Birmingham Archaeology Monograph Series 3

'Out of darkness, cometh light'

Life and Death in Nineteenth-Century Wolverhampton

Excavation of the overflow burial ground of St Peter's Collegiate Church, Wolverhampton 2001–2002

Josephine Adams
Kevin Colls

with contributions by

Iraia Arabaolaza, Lynne Bevan, Anthea Boylston, Gary Coates, Leonie Driver, Rowena Gale, Annette Hancocks, Emma Hancox, Erica Macey-Bracken, Charlotte Neilson, Paola Ponce, Stephanie Ratkái and Sarah Watt

Illustrations by Nigel Dodds and Kevin Colls

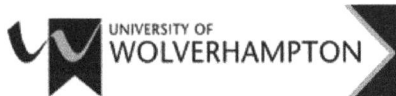

UNIVERSITY OF WOLVERHAMPTON

BAR British Series 442
2007

Published in 2016 by
BAR Publishing, Oxford

BAR British Series 442

Birmingham Archaeology Monograph Series 3

'Out of darkness, cometh light'
Life and Death in Nineteenth-Century Wolverhampton

ISBN 978 1 4073 0123 5

BAR Publishing is the trading name of British Archaeological Reports (Oxford) Ltd.
British Archaeological Reports was first incorporated in 1974 to publish the BAR
Series, International and British. In 1992 Hadrian Books Ltd became part of the BAR
group. This volume was originally published by Archaeopress in conjunction with
British Archaeological Reports (Oxford) Ltd / Hadrian Books Ltd, the Series principal
publisher, in 2007. This present volume is published by BAR Publishing, 2016.

Printed in England

BAR
PUBLISHING

BAR titles are available from:

BAR Publishing
122 Banbury Rd, Oxford, OX2 7BP, UK
EMAIL   info@barpublishing.com
PHONE   +44 (0)1865 310431
FAX   +44 (0)1865 316916
www.barpublishing.com

Contents

List of Figures

List of Plates

List of Tables

Acknowledgements

The archaeological excavation of the overflow burial ground of St Peter's Church, Wolverhampton, was carried out by Birmingham University Field Archaeology Unit (now Birmingham Archaeology) for Thomas Vale Construction on behalf of the University of Wolverhampton. The post-excavation programme was undertaken on behalf of the University of Wolverhampton. Mike Shaw, the Black Country Archaeologist, monitored the excavations on behalf of Wolverhampton City Council.

The excavation was managed by Gary Coates and supervised by Charlotte Neilson, assisted by Bob Bracken and carried out by Kate Bain, Suzy Blake, Alison Dingle, Mary Duncan, Nathan Flavell, Rebecca Hardy, Maurice Hopper, Richard Lee, Helen Martin, Emily Murray, David Priestley, Barrie Simpson, James Taylor and Steve Williams. The processing of artefacts and human remains was supervised by Erica Macey-Bracken and Emma Hancox, with the assistance of Lydia Bird, Alison Dingle, Rebeckah Judah, and David Priestley. The post-excavation programme was managed by Alex Jones and Josephine Adams. Editing was undertaken by Della Hooke and Amanda Forster. Thanks are due to Simon Buteux, Mike Shaw and Anthea Boylston for comments on the draft text.

Many thanks are due to the contractors, Thomas Vale Construction, especially Jonathan Davies, Don Roberts and Kevin Zamur for their co-operation, patience and assistance. Thanks are also due to J A Burke Construction, notably Patrick Durkin and Jim Burke, also Shaun Keating and Laurence Chambers.

Annette Hancocks would like to thank Roxanne Fea, Curator of the British Dental Association Museum for her assistance. The co-operation and assistance of Paul Adams, Mike Goodwin and Anthony Turner from the University of Wolverhampton was much appreciated. Thanks are also due to Kevin Grayson and Gill Dixon from Bond Bryan Architects, and to Gary Earle, Executive Officer, Coroners Section, Home Office, for his advice and assistance.

The illustrations were prepared by Nigel Dodds and Kevin Colls. The studio photography was by Graham Norrie.

Josephine Adams would like to thank the following: the staff of the Wolverhampton Archives and Local Studies, Stafford Records Office and Lichfield Diocesan Office; Sue Galloway for her analysis of the burial records and local knowledge; George Bolton, the verger of St Peter's Church; David Barker from the Stoke on Trent Archaeology Service; Iain Soden and Jenny Wakely for the unpublished report from Holy Trinity Church, Coventry which took place following the excavation at St Mary's Church, Coventry undertaken by Northamptonshire Archaeology in 1999-2000.

Iraia Arabaolaza and Paula Ponce are very grateful to the following members of the Biological Anthropology Research Centre, Anthea Boylston, Alan Ogden, Darlene Weston, Jo Buckberry and Christopher Knusel.

Summary

Between October 2001 and January 2002, Birmingham University Field Archaeology Unit (now Birmingham Archaeology) carried out archaeological excavations for Thomas Vale Construction (on behalf of the University of Wolverhampton) on the overflow burial ground of St Peter's Collegiate Church, Wolverhampton (NGR SO 3914 2989). The work was undertaken in advance of the construction of an extension to the Harrison Learning Centre.

The excavations revealed evidence of activity prior to the use of the area as a burial ground. Two pits and a gully were found, highly truncated, but may be associated with the grounds of a Deanery, which stood in this area during the medieval period.

The excavations recorded 152 human burials, dating to the mid-19th century. The majority of the burials were found with scant remains of wooden coffins and had been subject to the intercutting of graves and truncation by later building activity. Seven brick vaults were found, six of which had been emptied, probably during an earlier graveyard clearance. The intact vault and earth-cut burials were found in the southeastern part of the development site, which appeared not to have been cleared.

The preservation of human bone was generally good, despite the high levels of truncation. The sample provided a good opportunity for research into the health and lifestyles of the local population. Anthropological analysis was carried out on 150 skeletons, revealing some striking results. Of the individuals investigated, 42% died before the age of 20 and 76% of the sub-adults died before the age of five. An assessment of the pathology of the skeletons revealed a wide variety of diseases, conditions and trauma, including cases of tuberculosis, osteoarthritis, infectious diseases, syphilis, malignant tumours, and dental diseases. Three cases of amputations were also identified.

The archaeological evidence, scientific analysis of the skeletal remains, and the documentary research provide an important basis from which to reconstruct the lives and deaths of the people living in central Wolverhampton during the 19th century. The picture that emerges is that of a population largely suffering from bad health and poor living conditions and also employed in hazardous and stressful working environments. This picture of living and working conditions in an urban centre in the Victorian period is in sharp contrast to evidence recovered from a rural post-medieval burial group in Penn, Wolverhampton. The evidence from Penn, as well as data from excavations at St Martin's in Birmingham and Holy Trinity in Coventry, are compared to the results from this project, revealing yet more sharp contrasts in the age at death and pathology of the different populations.

The importance of post-medieval cemeteries, in particular their archaeological value, is still somewhat underrated. The authors hope this project will help to demonstrate the usefulness of such assemblages and the wealth of information that can be gleaned from archaeological, scientific, and documentary analysis.

CHAPTER 1

Project Background

Josephine Adams and Kevin Colls

INTRODUCTION

This volume documents the results of an archaeological excavation of the 19th-century overflow burial ground for St Peter's Collegiate Church, Wolverhampton (Fig 1). The fieldwork was carried out by Birmingham University Field Archaeology Unit (now Birmingham Archaeology) for Thomas Vale Construction on behalf of the University of Wolverhampton. It was required as part of a planning condition in advance of an extension to the Harrison Learning Centre at the University of Wolverhampton (NGR SO 3914 2989). The fieldwork took place between October 2001 and January 2002.

All archaeological work conformed to a brief prepared by Mike Shaw, Black Country Planning Archaeologist, Wolverhampton City Council (2001) and a written scheme of investigation prepared by Birmingham Archaeology (2001). The archaeological excavation and monitoring of groundworks adhered to the Home Office and Environmental Services regulations concerning the treatment and removal of human burials, under the provisions of the 1981 Disused Burials Act (Amendment). A risk assessment was also prepared by Birmingham Archaeology, prior to the commencement of excavation. A summary of results can also be found in the post excavation assessment (Coates and Nielson 2002).

From this point forward any reference to the burial ground of St Peter's will refer to the overflow graveyard associated with this project. Any reference to the churchyard of St Peter's shall refer to the graveyard immediately surrounding the church.

SITE LOCATION AND GEOLOGY

The development site lies to the north of St Peter's Church in Wolverhampton City Centre, within the Inner Ring Road (Fig 2). To the east and north is the Harrison Learning Centre, to the south is an access driveway, and to the west is St Peter's Square. The site had been raised above street level and contained mature trees, a grassed-over area and a covered walkway, which was built against the west wall of the Harrison Learning Centre (Plate 1).

Wolverhampton is on a spur of the Birmingham sandstone plateau. The area of the site is situated within the vicinity of the highest part of the plateau that slopes steeply towards the north and northwest. It is also part of a watershed for local drainage systems (Slater 1986, 35).

The drift geology consists of glacial clays, sands and gravels. Parts of this natural drift geology seem to have been heavily terraced in some areas of the University of Wolverhampton Campus development.

ARCHAEOLOGICAL BACKGROUND

St Peter's Church was reputedly founded by the Mercian royal family in the 7th century AD and was an important early Christian centre in the region. The area in which the development site now lies was, in the medieval and post-medieval periods, occupied by the Deanery of Wolverhampton and its associated grounds and gardens until 1819 when it was consecrated and used as an overflow burial ground for St Peter's. The southern section of the site was developed further in the early 20th century during the construction of St Peter's School and subsequent extensions. The overflow burial ground was futher cleared in 1973 during extension work to the University of Wolverhampton, including the clearance of most of the burial vaults.

An excavation carried out by Birmingham University Field Archaeology Unit in 1996 in an area to the east of the site uncovered a series of 19th-century brick-lined vaults in the northwestern corner of that site (SMR 8832; see Fig 2). This would correspond with the area most likely to have comprised the small part of the overflow burial ground enclosed within the School walls. Four skeletons were recovered stacked above each other in what probably constituted a family vault. The excavation also found that not all the uncovered vaults contained burials, and suggested that they may have been occupied and subsequently emptied prior to either the construction of the school or the 1973 development (Coates and Litherland 1996). However, no records could be found of this specific event. An 18th-century boundary wall, which probably delineated the eastern extent of the burial ground, was associated with one of the vaults, and incorporated a reused sandstone block which may originally have been associated with the medieval and post-medieval Deanery.

The excavation followed a desk-based assessment (Watt 2001), which reported that a clearance took place in 1973, but it was not known whether all or part of the site had been cleared. The report subsequently highlighted the possibility that human remains and burial vaults might be encountered. A series of test-pits across the development site prior to this excavation identified *in situ* articulated skeletons and burial vaults, albeit collapsed.

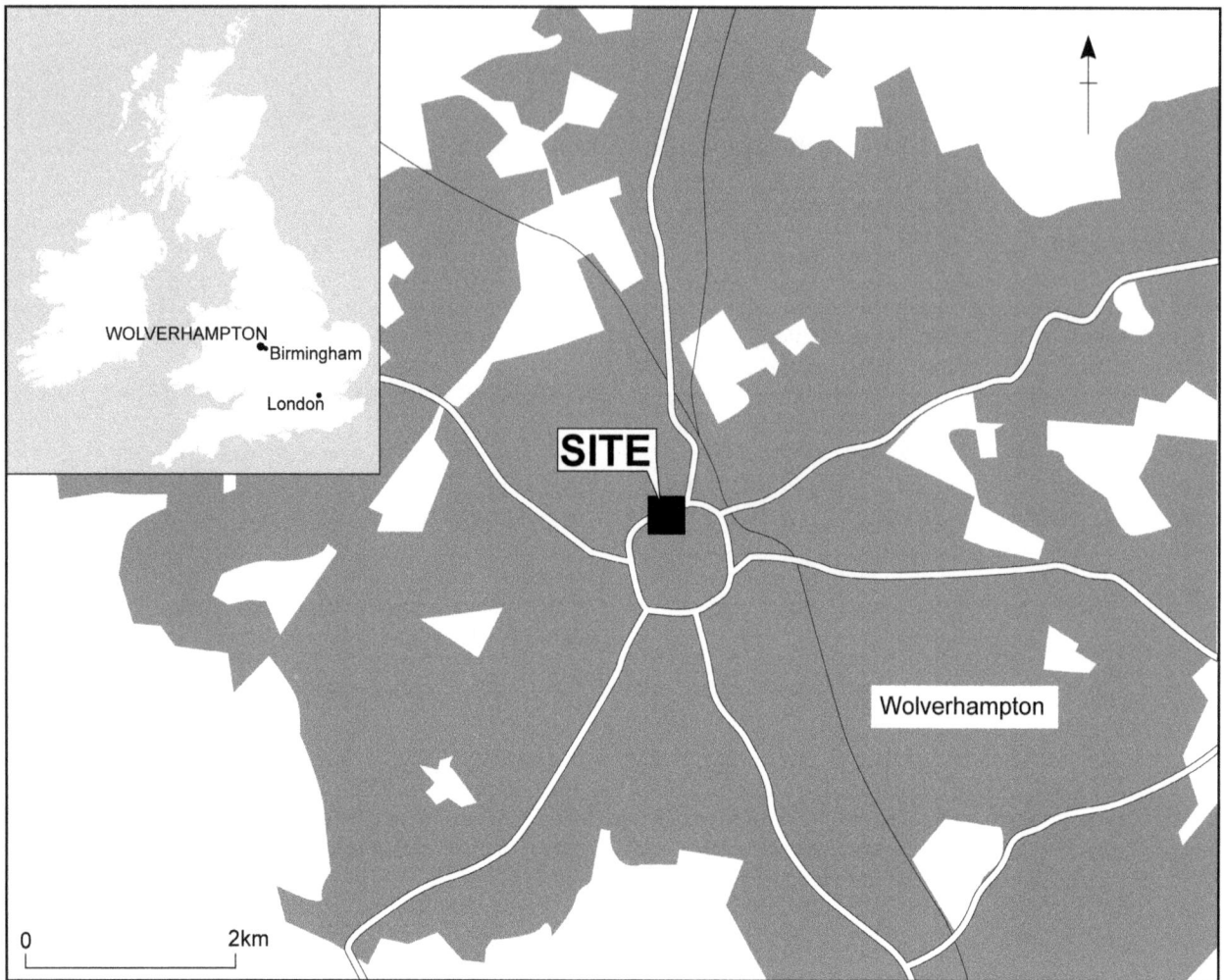

Figure 1   Site location plan

AIMS AND OBJECTIVES

The principal aim of the archaeological fieldwork was the excavation and recording of archaeological features, deposits and human burials that would be disturbed by the proposed development. The objectives and research aims were:

- To understand the occupation and utilisation of the site from the medieval period to the present.
- To identify and excavate any archaeological remains associated with the Deanery.
- To gain an understanding of the utilisation of the site as an overflow burial ground and to record and excavate any human remains, both articulated and disarticulated, that will be impacted by development.
- To record the structural elements of any burial vaults or lined graves encountered.
- To provide comparative material that will contribute to our understanding of the history of Wolverhampton.

More specifically, a research agenda was adopted to investigate the archaeological remains associated with the post-medieval burial ground. The key points of this research agenda were to:

- Undertake an anthropological study of the skeletons to assess the sex, stature, health, lifestyle and age of death of any individuals surviving as intact burials.
- Assess and compare the results of the study to other local post-medieval burial grounds.
- If possible, identify by name individuals buried in the burial ground and investigate aspects of their life, eg family history, occupation, residency, etc.
- Use any information gained to contribute to the wider picture of life, death and industry in Wolverhampton during the 19th century.
- Assess the archaeological and osteological importance of the skeletal assemblage on both a local and national scale.
- Assess the overall success of this approach to the investigation of post-medieval cemeteries.

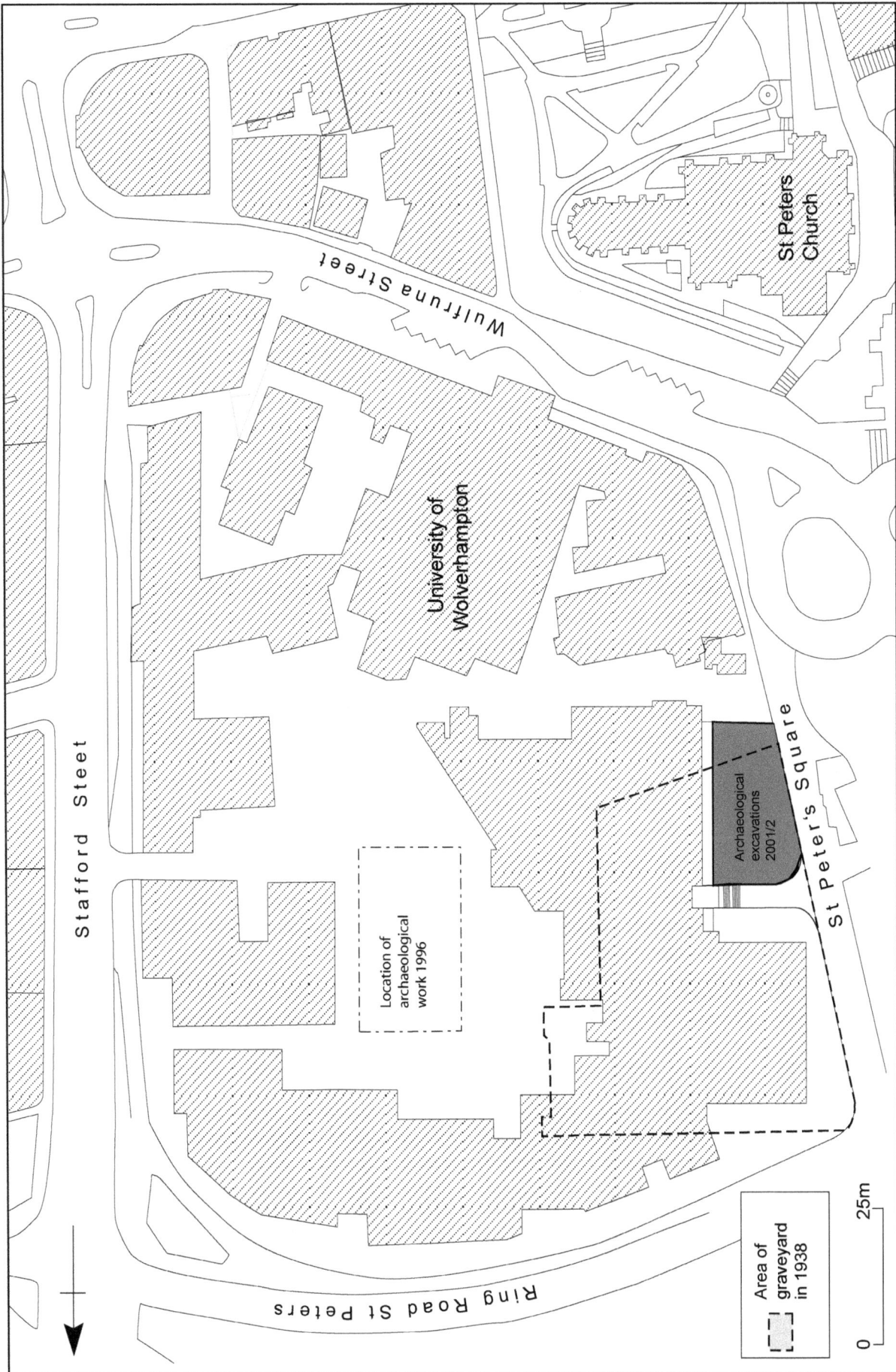

Figure 2   Excavation area

St Peters Church

Wulfruna Street

University of Wolverhampton

Stafford Steet

Ring Road St Peters

Location of archaeological work 1996

Archaeological excavations 2001/2

St Peter's Square

Area of graveyard in 1938

0   25m

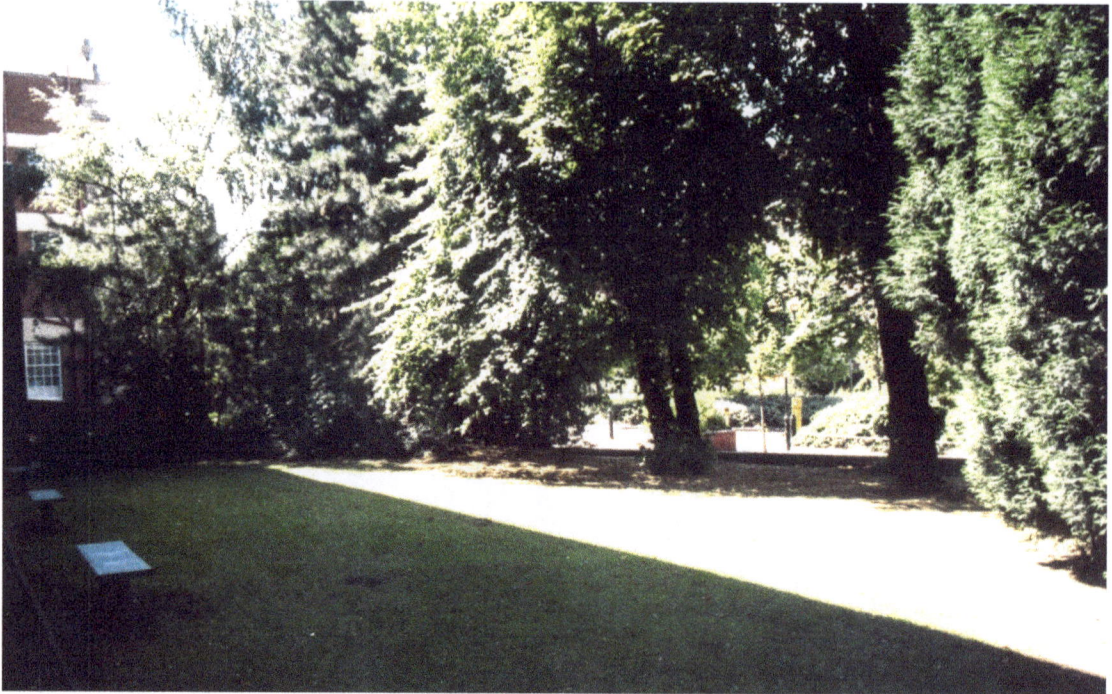

Plate 1   Area prior to fieldwork

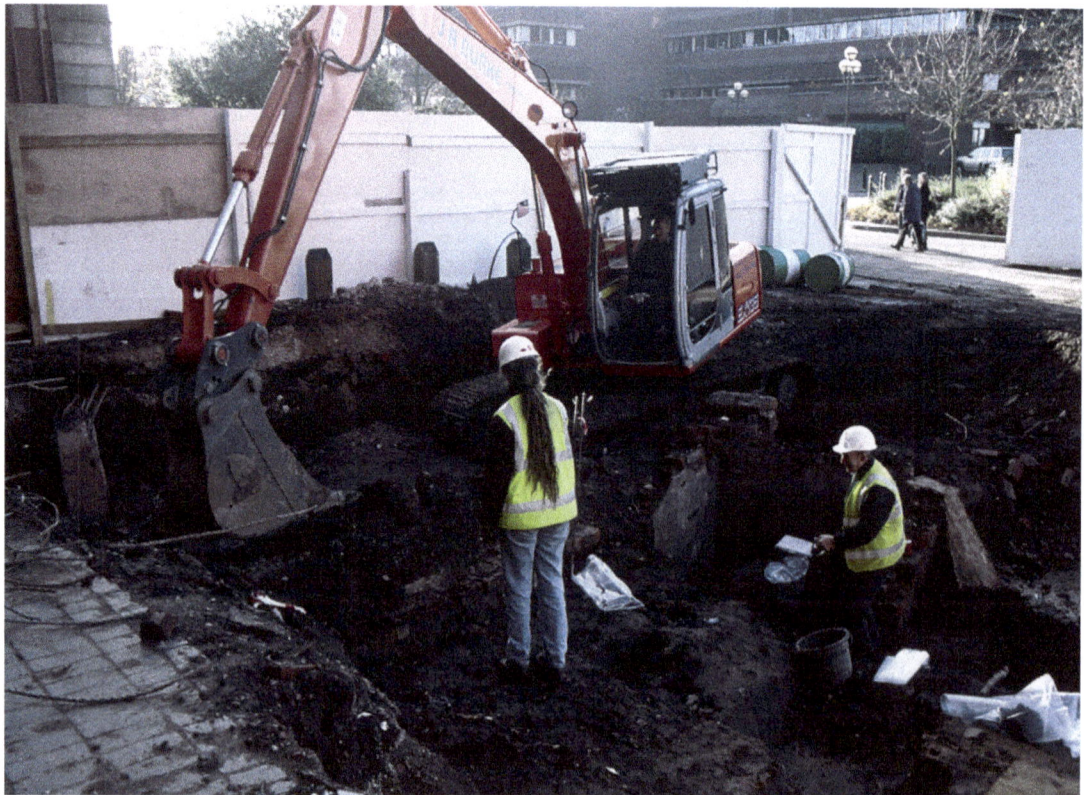

Plate 2   Excavation in progress

METHODOLOGY

Excavation

Over time, a considerable depth of overburden had accumulated over the archaeological deposits (Plate 1). This was removed using a mechanical excavator to the top of the uppermost archaeological horizon (Plate 2). A qualified archaeologist monitored this phase of works and recovered any disarticulated human bones or grave memorial fragments from the spoil. After the excavation, the groundworks associated with the new building were also monitored to record/ recover any isolated features or burials.

All the archaeological features and burials were recorded on a series of pro-forma sheets designed for on-site recording of contexts, features, skeletons, vaults, and grave memorials. A full drawn and photographic record was made to accompany the written record.

Burials

Articulated burials were manually excavated and recorded, and subsequently lifted. Infants and neonates, which were too delicate for on-site excavation, were removed as a complete sample and processed in the laboratory. Any objects associated with the burials were recorded and retrieved. Fragments of grave memorials were fully recorded and photographed and subsequently reburied on site.

The earth-cut graves were difficult to define as the site had been redeveloped a number of times since the burial ground had fallen into disuse. Graves cutting the natural clay were clear, but less so were the graves cutting through the subsoil. A number of burials were encountered running beneath the Learning Centre itself. As this building was constructed using piles, the skeletal remains close to the walls survived intact. These remains were excavated, with every attempt made to remove all of the bones that ran underneath the building.

Vaults

The vaults were excavated as individual features. The backfill in each vault was removed by hand or by mechanical excavator under supervision. Disarticulated and articulated bone was treated as discussed above. The vault structures were recorded, drawn and photographed.

Skeletal analysis

A detailed anthropological study of the articulated human remains was undertaken by the Biological Anthropology Research Centre, Department of Archaeological Sciences, University of Bradford. The full methodology for skeletal analysis is detailed in Chapter 5.

Documentary research

The historical research focused upon the names discovered on the grave memorials and *depositum* plates identified during the excavation. In most cases the information was incomplete, having been worn away or damaged over time, but where possible the name and date of death enabled some information to be discovered about each family. Only two *depositum* plates were recovered *in situ* from earth-cut burials.

Initially, the St Peter's burial records were examined but, whilst in the majority of cases this provides a list of everyone who was buried or had a funeral service at the church, it does not differentiate between those buried immediately around the church and those in the overflow burial ground.

The census returns for 1841, 1851, 1861 and 1871 were consulted, providing information about addresses, occupations and other family members. The 1792 Rates return was also studied, together with the St Catherine's Index (SCI), a national index that lists all births, deaths and marriages since 1837. Three death certificates were also studied in an effort to ascertain the cause of death of the individual and information about other family members. The local trade directories, which catalogue people either alphabetically or by their profession, provided information about individual's occupations, businesses or residential addresses. These directories are available from the late 18th century, but the coverage is not always complete, and in some cases inclusion may depend upon the individual's ability to pay for an entry. The International Genealogical Index (IGI), a county index of parish registers compiled by the Church of Jesus Christ of Latter Day Saints, which is available on fiche or online, was consulted, together with the National Burial Index (NGI), but in both cases coverage of Staffordshire is incomplete so they did not contribute much additional information.

The majority of this research was carried out using facilities at the Wolverhampton Archives and Local Studies.

CHAPTER 2

The Parish, the Church and the Burial Grounds

Josephine Adams and Leonie Driver

HISTORY OF WOLVERHAMPTON
by Josephine Adams

The earliest mention of Wolverhampton comes in AD 985 when an area of land at 'Hampton' was granted by King Æthelred to Wulfrun, a Mercian noblewoman. Part of this land she in turn granted in AD 994 to the church at Wolverhampton (Hooke 1986, 16–26). The earliest known linkage of the name of the settlement and its benefactor comes in the 1070s when the church at *Wulvrenehamptonia* was granted by William the Conqueror to Samson, his chaplain and, later, Bishop of Worcester. In the Domesday Survey of 1086 the priests of the church at *Hantone* are said to hold 1ha of land here from Samson. On the estate there were six villeins and 30 bordars, together with 14 slaves. With dependents this would suggest a population of around 200, but the church holding was only part of the settlement. There was also a royal manor which is not mentioned in Domesday Book (Slater 1986, 29).

By 1180 a regular market took place in the town, an act formalised in 1258 with the granting of a charter by King Henry III to the Dean of Wolverhampton to hold an annual fair and a weekly market every Wednesday. Despite suffering an outbreak of the plague in the 14th century, the town flourished, and the next 100 years saw the development of the woollen trade. Raw wool from the nearby Welsh Marches was spun into yarn and woven into cloth in the town (Mander and Tildesley 1960, 35). Many local families, notably the Levesons, the Ridleys and the Cresswells, became very wealthy from this trade and some reinvested their money into improving the town. This resulted in, amongst other projects, the church being largely rebuilt and the establishment of a grammar school (www.wlv.ac.uk/~in2021/oldwlv).

As the town grew in size, there was an increasing threat of fire resulting from the greater concentration of timber, plaster and thatch houses – all of which burnt easily. Major fires were recorded in 1590 and 1696, destroying a large number of houses and leaving many of the town's residents homeless (Mander and Tildesley 1960, 60).

The 16th century saw the discovery of coal and ironstone locally and this was to transform the area (Mander and Tildesley 1960, 143). Many small ironworking businesses developed and the town became well known for the numerous small items that were produced. During the Civil War many ironmasters profited by making arms and ordnance, doubtless for both sides (*ibid* 1960, 82).

However, it was the growth of the lock industry that was to dominate the local economy in the 17th century, with locks and keys produced as early as 1603. In 1686, Dr Plot, in his *Natural History of Staffordshire*, noted 'the act of lock making to be far advanced towards perfection' (Mander and Tildesley 1960, 106), and this lock-making tradition continued in the area, although the focus for this industry was later to shift to nearby Willenhall (*ibid*, 144). The 1770 Trade Directory lists 118 lock makers in the town, but of almost equal importance, with 116 names, was the production of buckles. The directory also lists 30 steel toy makers, who produced ornamental buckles, sword hilts and jewellery made of burnished steel. This jewellery became very fashionable, and became more and more elaborate, often decorated with marcasite and semi-precious stones. Up to the early 1790s this jewellery was in great demand but gradually it became less fashionable, and this, together with the cheaper production methods developed in nearby Birmingham, signalled the demise of the industry in Wolverhampton (*ibid*, 145).

Another trade that developed in the 18th century from the tin-plate industry was the art of japanning. This involved painting and lacquering the steel and then varnishing it to produce highly elaborate, colourful designs that were used to cover all kinds of domestic equipment. Papier mâché products were also made and japanned in the same way as the tin-plate ware (Mander and Tildesley 1960, 145). As a result of the demand for varnish to supply the japanning trade, the Mander brothers, John and Benjamin, started a paint and varnish factory that was to become another important facet of the town's industrial diversity (*ibid*).

During the 19th century, industrialisation continued, and the lure of employment attracted immigrants to the town, not only from outlying rural areas but also from Wales and Ireland. As production methods improved, the emphasis changed from small-scale manufacture to heavier forms of engineering with bicycles, cars, lorries and buses soon being produced (www.localhistory.scit.wlv.ac.uk). After the 1832 Reform Act, Wolverhampton was granted two parliamentary seats and in 1848 it became a borough. The Council then took over from the Town Commissioners and public services, education and housing were improved.

During the 20th century, Wolverhampton continued to expand, with immigration from Italy and Poland, and later from Africa and the Caribbean, contributing to its diverse culture. In 1992 the Polytechnic, having merged with several other local colleges, achieved University status, and in 2001 the borough was granted city status.

THE TOWN IN THE EARLY 19TH CENTURY
by Josephine Adams

The 19th century was a time of unprecedented change in England as the effects of industrialisation spread across the country. Wolverhampton was already a manufacturing centre and in 1750 was said to have a population of 7,454 people living in 1,440 houses (Taylor's map of Wolverhampton). Nevertheless the 19th century saw an ever-increasing pattern of growth. The existence of a rich coalfield, together with supplies of iron ore and fire clay immediately to the east of the town, fuelled this growth as Wolverhampton benefited from its location as one of the major towns of the area which became known as the 'The Black Country' (www.localhistory.scit.wlv.ac.uk). The population increased exponentially from 12,565 at the start of the century to 94,187 at the end, a 750% increase, as people migrated from the country attracted by the promise of work in the new industries (Table 1).

The population of the Black Country as a whole grew much faster in the first half of the century than that of the rest of the country, reflecting the rapid growth of the area as the new industrial processes took hold. Illustrative of the changes in the nature of employment in the area, in 1801 26% of the population was engaged in trade but by 1881 this figure had risen to 57% (Barnsby 1980, 12 and 19).

The presence of the coal seam was the most important factor in the development of the area. The coal was near the surface, so the pits were shallow, small and typically employed only a few men in each. In 1874 nearly 37,000 miners were employed at 469 collieries, an average of less than 80 per colliery. This small-scale production resulted in an organisational structure that was peculiar to the Black Country (Barnsby 1980, 24), with many of these small concerns run by sub-contractors or 'butties' who were only concerned with making money and cared little for the safety of their employees. For the miners it was a precarious occupation, since the method of extraction involved workers, called pikemen, undermining a section of the coal-face leaving only a very thin rib, called a spern, to support the roof (Fig 3). When the undercutting had progressed far enough, they worked on scaffolding cutting a channel upwards to loosen the roof. This was then brought down by long-handled picks, called prickers, resulting in the coal falling

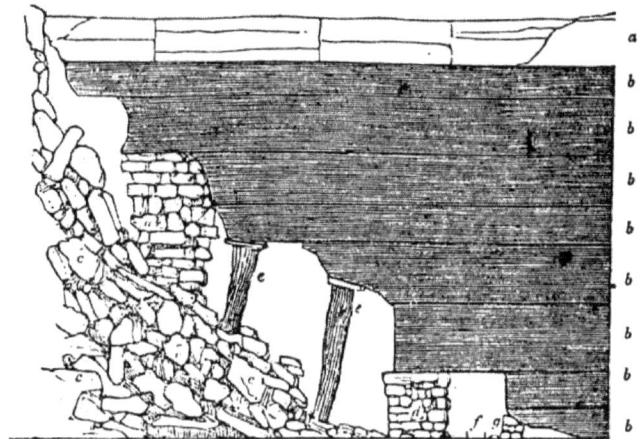

Plan of working the thick Coal at Shutt End Colliery.

a. The Measures above the Coal.
b, b, b, &c. The various beds of the 10-yard Coal.
c, c, c, &c. The Spoil (or broken measures) which falls down as the Coal is got out.
d, d, and g. Cogs built of this Spoil to support the Coal.
e, e. Timber put up for the same purpose.
f. The Railroad, which is carried forwards as the work advances towards the right hand.

Figure 3   Diagram showing method of coal extraction

from the roof. Much of the coal was broken and unusable; the whole process was very dangerous and fatalities were common. The thin coal and ironstone mines were less dangerous to work in but the wages were lower. In addition, the only lighting was from candles that increased the risk of explosion (Robson 2002, 24).

Unlike the textile or mining centres of the north, Wolverhampton and the surrounding areas were not dependent upon a single product. However, many were related to the iron industry, so any fluctuation in the trade had a marked effect on local economy (Robson 2002, 22). Products produced in the area included locks, edge tools, cut nails, screws, springs, fenders, hollow ware, papier mâché and japanware.

At the beginning of the century there were few large factories; instead the work was focused in small-scale industrial units or workshops, often in back yards or even within the workers' homes. The 1802 Rate Book clearly illustrates the domination of the locksmith, with 162 establishments listed, followed by 48 buckle makers. Other occupations included hinge makers, key makers, snuffer makers and steel toy makers (Roper 1969, 5ff). The reason for this prevalence of small businesses, like the domestic nailers and locksmiths, could be attributed in part to the fact that they did not require a large initial outlay or a big workforce, so were relatively easy to establish. In many cases a composite operation was broken down into its component parts, each small enough

Table 1 Population increase 1801–1901 (Source: Mitchell and Deane 1962)

1801	1811	1821	1831	1841	1851	1861	1871	1881	1891	1901
12565	14836	18380	24732	36382	49985	60860	68291	75766	82662	94187

to be carried out separately in small workshops where the individual could work at his own speed. The saddle and harness industry in nearby Walsall and Bloxwich was an example of this, with many items being made in small workshops employing no more than six workers (Robson 2002, 26). This domestic outworking in such trades as nailing, chain making, jewellery and button making was to survive in the area long after it had ceased elsewhere. Eventually however, as the century progressed and mechanisation increased, these small workshops began to suffer, notably affecting the nail-making fraternity whose already precarious livelihood was threatened by machines that could, as a contemporary commentator said, make 'nails of an excellent quality by pressure, and they are turned out of a machine like flour from a mill' (James Boydell, quoted in Robson 2002, 22).

During this time of unprecedented growth, at the end of the 18th and beginning of the 19th centuries, the rapid increase in population highlighted the need for some form of local government to combat the increasing social problems. Most Black Country towns had, up to then, been governed by ineffectual manorial courts but in 1779 Wolverhampton became the first town in the area to obtain an Improvement Act (Barnsby 1980, 54). In this Act it is stated that Wolverhampton was a 'large, populous, and trading town' and that many of its streets 'are narrow and incommodious for Passengers and Carriages' (quoted in Mander and Tildesley 1960, 138). As a result, through the efforts of the Commissioners who were appointed to put the Act into effect, many buildings were demolished, streets were paved and streetlights installed. However, these improvements were largely confined to the town centre, where the main consideration seemed to be to facilitate improved transport and commerce rather than to improve the health of the population (Barnsby 1980, 54). In 1814 a new Act was passed that increased the power of the Commissioners, an unelected group of local businessmen whose own interests may have been paramount, and in 1837 the Poor Law Union was formed. By 1832, when the town was affected by cholera, it became apparent that these groups were unable to cope with a town the size of Wolverhampton, but it was not until 1848 that it became a borough and the commissioners were deprived of their power (Mander and Tildesley 1960, 139; Barnsby 1980, 54).

By 1788 the number of houses in the town had risen to 2,270, an increase of 58% on the 1750 figure, many being squeezed into gaps in the existing courts. The absence of building regulations meant that in the ensuing years houses built round a central courtyard and in narrow alleys were crammed in at the highest possible density, the results of which were to become the source of many problems (Barnsby 1987, 6). The Children's Employment Commission of 1843 describes the working-class areas of the town as like a 'rabbit warren', with narrow passages between the houses leading to small courts with 'houses, hutches or hovels' leading off them. These in turn had other passages leading to unpaved yards and blind alleys. The problems were exacerbated by the presence of the many workshops, the majority of which were at the back of the houses. These workshops were connected by passages that apparently originated from the householders in the street retaining a right of way alongside their houses to go to their workshops. Subsequently, other small rooms could be built over these workshops to be utilised by another workshop, or occupied by even more families. The houses themselves are described as 'indifferent, bare of all comfort', squalid and dirty with very little furniture. Livestock such as horses, donkeys and pigs were often driven through the narrow lanes, producing a 'deep sludge' that had to be scraped to one side, and stagnant pools that gathered in any small hollow (Children's Employment Commission). The state of the streets even moved one visitor to the town to write to the *Wolverhampton Chronicle* on July 26th 1843, saying;

To the Editor,
Sir,
….I have been in most of the large towns in England, and at many on the continent, and nowhere have I seen anything so disgustingly filthy as the state of Wolverhampton appeared this morning. It would seem that the streets are considered common dunghill-heaps of filth, of decayed vegetables, of ashes, the sweepings of shops, and other offensive matter, meet the pedestrian at every turn. If the daily occurrence of such nuisances has benumbed the feelings of the inhabitants, perhaps the astonishment which such a state of their town strikes a stranger may awaken them to some sense of its uncleanliness.

Your's obediently,
VIATOR

The water supply and sanitation facilities were also inadequate in the growing town, although the Children's Employment Commission pointed out that many houses were 'built on a little elevation sloping towards the passage' and 'where these spaces are large enough to admit of it, there is generally a pump in the middle, the handle of which as it rises is sometimes in danger of breaking a window behind, while the spout fills the hovel in front if the door be not closed' (Children's Employment Commission).

To ameliorate the problem many wells were dug, either to serve the public or in private houses, and these were to be the main source of water until 1844 when the Wolverhampton Waterworks Company was founded. However, this was not the end of the problem and the supply of an adequate water supply to the town continued to be problematic for many years to come (Barnsby 1980, 79).

Very few of these houses had underground drainage or lavatories, although some of the better courts had a communal lavatory that many people would use. The correspondent cited above also addressed this absence of sanitary facilities in his postscript:

P.S. I am told that there are literally some thousands of small houses in Wolverhampton (many of them belonging to rich individuals) without drains, privies or ash-holes! Well may all respectable people think it time for the government to interpose the strong arm of the law, and compel such persons to provide conveniences for houses from which the most extortionate rents are wrung.

However, despite adverse reports in 1843 from R A Slaney Esq, one of Her Majesty's Commissioners, it seems little was done to improve conditions in the town, and in 1848 the state of the town was discussed again by W A Lewis in a lecture given at the Wolverhampton Athenaeum and reported in the Wolverhampton Chronicle of 26th January 1848. He equated the high death rate in the town to murder, noting that there had been a particularly high rate of deaths in comparison with other towns during 1848. Lewis also cited the usual problems of inadequate drainage, lack of clean water supply and overcrowded housing, in particular the high number of Irish immigrants who crowded into two-bedroom lodging houses. He also stated that pigs should not be kept in sties near houses, slaughter houses should not be built within the town and that 'contamination of the atmosphere by churchyards' was a problem. Lewis also felt that 'typhus fever always begins among the poor, in the most unhealthy localities in the town. After it has done its worst among the victims of poverty and dirt it attacks the middle classes'; he added that 'it never originates among the wealthier classes, but finds its way there after having been fatal in the worst parts of the town'.

Lewis concluded his lecture by alluding to the fact that the high death rate in the town, that he attributed in part to poor living conditions, could also be accounted for by the difficult and dangerous occupations in which many people in the area were involved, in particular, ironworkers and 'colliers working half their labours under ground with their health previously debilitated having commenced their life as mere children'.

As if to prove Lewis's point about the unhealthy conditions of the town, one of the Magistrates reports in the same paper that someone had been summoned for non-payment of highway rates. The defendant replied that he had no objection to the rate, but he wanted to appear before the Magistrate to complain about the dreadful condition of the street in which he lived: 'Southampton Street', he said, 'was the dirtiest street in Wolverhampton'. The Magistrate told him he would have to take his complaint to the Commissioners.

The problem of overcrowded churchyards mentioned by Lewis was not peculiar to Wolverhampton. Throughout the country, as population increased, the urban churchyards were unable to cope with the demand for space. There was a growing awareness that this overcrowding added to the unsanitary conditions in towns where public health facilities were already inadequate.

Subsequently, a Sanitary Report in the *Wolverhampton Chronicle* of 9th February 1848 reported that Dr Dehane from the Board of Guardians stated that it was the intention of Her Majesty's government to introduce remedial measures as soon as possible to address the 'defective sanitary condition of populous towns'.

The Rawlinson Report of 1849 states that because of the natural elevation of Wolverhampton, sewers and drains could have been constructed quite cheaply. However, because of the lack of town planning this had not happened. There was no central organisation of the construction of the sewers. Some had been constructed at public expense, while others had been dug by private individuals, resulting in no common drainage connections. In one case, the sewerage near St John's Square had percolated through the graveyard into the wells of the houses near by (Rawlinson 1849, 19). In addition, where drains existed, they were also inadequate and often too near the surface. E H Coleman, a surgeon of the town stated that:

In the worse drained and most crowded portions of the town fever most frequently prevailed, there were districts of the town where fever was unknown, and there were other places where it was rarely absent, and in those parts there were no drains. When the cholera visited the town in 1832, it prevailed in all those places where fever was common (Rawlinson 1849, 19).

As compulsory recording of all births and deaths did not begin until April of 1837, it is not possible to obtain accurate death rates prior to that year. However, from 1840 until 1870 the Registrar General published birth and death rates in ten-year periods. A comparison of all the Black Country towns between 1840 and 1870, in which Wolverhampton is split into east and west districts, clearly shows that the eastern part of the town had the highest death rate in the area (Table 2). The difference between the working-class area, in the east, and the wealthier western section of the town is clearly illustrated. The table also illustrates that Wolverhampton east had a much higher death rate than the average for the rest of the country.

Endemic diseases at the time included tuberculosis, typhoid, scarlet fever, measles, and various forms of pneumonia (Kunitz in Kiple 1993, 289). Mr Lewis, quoted above, suggests that the people of Wolverhampton, previously 'debilitated by improper and insufficient food', were also 'living in a very impure and poisoned atmosphere' which resulted in them being weak and unable to fight off infection. He states that in 1847 typhus killed many parents, while many of their children died of scarlet fever (*Wolverhampton Chronicle* 26th

Table 2 Death rates in Wolverhampton 1840–1870, deaths per 1000 population (Source: Barnsby 1980, 61-63)

	1841-1850	1851-1860	1861-1870
Wolverhampton east	32.0	33.1	29.9
Wolverhampton west	21.3	23.0	20.6
Black Country	25.7	26.2	24.3
England & Wales	22.4	22.2	22.5

January 1848). According to the 1843 report of the Children's Employment Commission, asthma was prevalent amongst locksmiths and colliers, although this may be an all-encompassing term that covers all types of chest infection. In the early 19th century, pulmonary tuberculosis was the most common cause of death in the newly emerging urban centres (Aufderheide and Rodriguez Martin 1998, 130). So, with the aforementioned poor housing and inadequate ventilation in the narrow streets, it is likely that many of the people of the town suffered from the condition. One skeleton from the excavations (HB 40) showed spine lesions compatible with tuberculosis (see Chapter 5).

Syphilis had become a significant problem by this time, although the term had only come into use towards the end of the 18th century, and other symptoms may have been mistakenly attributed to the illness (Arrizabalaga in Kiple 1993, 1025). It is likely that syphilis was a problem in the town, as in many other urban centres, and this was supported by strong evidence of the disease in two of the burials (HB 44 and HB 75). The contemporary treatment involved the application of mercury (Roberts and Cox 2003, 340), which was found associated with another burial (HB 140), a fact that, to a degree, may be the evidence for its presence (see Chapter 7). In the 1802 Rate Book a prostitute named 'Martha' was listed at 87 Bilston Street, indicating perhaps, the tolerant attitude towards prostitution. This was to change by the 1860s, when prostitution became a cause of concern to government, the church, philanthropists and feminists. The problem, considered by many to be 'a social evil', was addressed by a variety of methods including government intervention, in the form of the Contagious Diseases Acts, the first of which was passed in 1864 (Bartley 1996, 78).

Poor diet combined with overcrowded living conditions in the dark narrow streets and alleyways resulted in vitamin deficiency related conditions, especially in the children. The 1843 Children's Employment Commission highlighted the problem of poor diet, stating that 'the quality of the food is not good, bad meat is continually sold in the markets, and the children are frequently fed on red herrings, or potatoes, or bread with lard upon it, for their dinners – and have not always sufficient even of this'.

Rickets, a condition involving skeletal deformity and growth problems in children, can be attributed to a lack of vitamin D that is obtained, in part, from sunlight.

Significantly the British Medical Journal of 1889 highlighted 'the coalfield of the Black Country' as having a high prevalence of the disease (Owen 1889). Rickets could affect the pelvis (Roberts and Cox 2003, 309) and may have contributed to high maternal and infant death rates in the town. In addition, a diet that lacks fresh fruit and vegetables may be deficient in vitamin C, resulting in scurvy, a problem that also affected bone and dental development. The Children's Employment Commission of 1843 describes some children as 'delicate, some sickly, many ill-formed, meagre, and awry (or even with incipient malformations), some badly deformed and in stature they are stunted', all clear illustrations that the poor diet that could result in rickets and scurvy affected them. The skeletal analysis produced evidence of both conditions together with osteomalacia, which results from deficiency of vitamin D in adulthood (see Chapter 5).

The increasing concern about the health of the children of the town was highlighted again in 1848 when, as a result of the Public Health Act, a government inspector visited the town and reported that one in six children died in their first year and that life expectancy at birth was only just over 19 years. This is confirmed by the skeletal report (see Chapter 5) which shows that, in the sample from St Peter's, infant mortality, especially in the weaning group, was 40% and the highest percentage of the human burials examined was in the under-18 category. The evidence of *cribra orbitalia* is also high, the explanation for which could again be the poor diet that infants received. Some contemporary feeding practices included feeding infants 'pap' or 'panada', a mixture of flour and water which, as well as being nutritionally inadequate, was often prepared in unhygienic surroundings, increasing the risk of gastric infection (Roberts and Cox 2003, 307). The Children's Employment Commission Report of 1843 also attributed the high death rate in infants to the custom of administering Godfrey's Cordial to infants and young children to keep them quiet or 'sleeping them' while their parents were out at work. This was a mixture of boiled treacle, water and a dose of opium made by the local chemist or his wife, the ingredients of which were not always precisely calculated. This could result in varying amounts of opium being administered to the child, often while the mother was out at work. The report states that 'many children are killed by it. Some waste away to skeletons, and their sufferings are prolonged; other died more easily'.

A disease that was to affect the town several times in the early 19th century was cholera, an acute infectious disease that spread to Europe from the Indian subcontinent in the early 1800s. There were major outbreaks of the disease in Britain in 1832, 1849, 1853–4 and 1856, and Wolverhampton was affected on each occasion. In 1832 the town escaped lightly with only 193 deaths, in comparison with nearby Bilston that lost 741 people. However, in 1849 500 people died. The epidemics highlighted the inadequacies of the medical facilities in the town. During the 1832 outbreak those who were able to pay went to the Dispensary in Queen Street, while some free treatment was available at the Medical Hall and Vapour Bath in Dudley Street as long as the claimant could provide a letter from a respectable person saying that they could not pay. By 1849 the South Staffordshire General Hospital had been built but it refused to accept any cholera patients, preferring to isolate them in the workhouse or in specially erected tents on Goldthorn Hill, two miles out of town (www.scit.wlv.ac.uk.local/victorian).

It is impossible to know how many of the people buried in St Peter's were victims of cholera since it has no effect on the skeleton. Indeed one of the characteristics of the disease was the speed with which it affected the victim, with death often occurring within hours of the first symptoms manifesting themselves. It was not until the 1850s that the cause of the disease was linked to contaminated water supplies. Its appearance before then was considered to be God's punishment for sinful behaviour, or as a result of miasma, poisonous gases allegedly that had been generated by filth (Roberts and Cox 2003, 337). In nearby Bilston, the blame was firmly attributed to the presence of the many immigrants in the town, whose bad behaviour was likened to that of the Israelites in the Bible (Price 1832, 18). This ignorance about the causes of the disease led to doctors mistakenly prescribing bleeding, blistering or cupping to the sufferers, or even prescribing milk (www.swan.ac.uk/teaching). Other remedies were advertised in the *Staffordshire Advertiser* in 1832, amongst them was the application of lime, produced by a local company, and anti-cholera brandy, and the dashing of the stomach and bowels with cold water. However, gradually, the realisation that the unsanitary conditions that existed in the town were a major contributory factor led to an improvement in public health facilities.

The cholera epidemics also increased the pressure on local churchyards. Up to 1849 there were only three Anglican graveyards in Wolverhampton, at St Peter's Collegiate Church, St John's, and St George's, together with a Roman Catholic burial ground in North Street. St George's was used predominantly for cholera victims, with graves being dug 20 feet deep to accommodate as many bodies as possible (www.scit.wlv.ac.uk.local/victorian). The bodies of the deceased were buried as soon as possible after death, the burials often taking place at night to alleviate panic (Robson 2002, 126).

As well as fatalities amongst the population that could be attributed to public health, accidents were a major cause of death. The Children's Employment Commission (Mitchell: 1st Report Mines 1842) reported deaths (not only relating to children) associated with fire, drowning, murder, suicide (although suicide victims would not be given a Christian burial), and accidents associated with horses, wagons and gigs, and falls from ladders. In addition the report provided details of deaths associated with the mining industry that included falls associated with coal shafts, deaths from falling coal, clods and rubbish, drowning, suffocation, and explosion. There were also accidents at ironstone pits, ironworks and lime works. Notably in Wolverhampton two lads aged twelve and 17 fell to their death down an ironstone pit shaft and a ten year old was drawn between the cop-wheels of a steam-engine at an ironworks (*ibid.*, 14–16). The use of child labour was regulated in 1842 when an Act of Parliament forbade the employment of women and children under ten for work underground, although those already employed were allowed to remain. In practice this did not affect the women of Wolverhampton because none had ever been employed in the Black Country coalfields (Barnsby 1980, 28).

In the early part of the 19th century, leisure pursuits in the town included dog fighting, cock fighting and bull baiting, which, since they were banned in the 1777 Town Act, were held just outside the town boundary at Chapel Ash. Pugilism or bare-knuckle boxing was also popular. This dates from the 18th century and fights were fought in un-timed rounds that only ended when one contestant was knocked down (www.tiscali.co.uk/reference/ encyclopaedia/hutchinson). This often resulted in broken hands, wrists and noses and could account for some of the fractures found in the burial ground. In particular, three men (HB 56, HB 120, HB 130) had well-healed fractures in some metacarpal bones, and one (HB 120) also had fractured both nasal bones at some time in his life, an indication, perhaps, that he had been involved in the sport. A local boxer, William Perry, known as the Tipton Slasher, was to become world bare-knuckle boxing world champion from 1850–1857, an indication of the popularity of the sport in the area (www.tiscali/ myweb.co.uk/poetrypages/photo).

Other fractures revealed in the skeletal sample on ribs or sternum, for example, may have been caused by some degree of interpersonal violence, industrial injury or accident in the over-crowded streets.

There were three examples of amputations in the sample (Chapter 5), which are significant in that they illustrate that this medical procedure was being carried out at this time. Another amputee, of a similar date, discovered in Birmingham, corroborates this. The Birmingham skeleton showed evidence of some healing after the operation but died shortly afterwards, almost certainly from an infection introduced during the operation (Brickley, in Krakowicz and Rudge 2002, 18–19). The three from the

Wolverhampton sample also showed evidence of healing and therefore survival after the operation, but it is impossible to know how long they lived after the operation. This was a high-risk procedure at the time because of the danger of haemorrhage, shock and sepis, and mortality rates of 60% were recorded. It was not until the discovery of chloroform in the mid-19th century and carbolic spray in the 1870s that survival rates improved (Roberts and Cox 2003, 313–15). When the local hospital opened in 1849 there was one consulting surgeon, three surgeons and one house surgeon listed amongst the staff. In 1847, Mr Edward Hayling Coleman, the house surgeon, carried out the third ever operation recorded in England using anaesthesia, a factor that may have aided the recovery of the amputees (www.localhistory.scit.wlv.ac.uk/articles/RoyalHospital).

In 1825 a racecourse was built to the west of the town, where racing continued until 1878 when the land became a public park (Mander and Tildesley 1960, 164–5). The tradition of St Monday, in which workers took the day off, was prevalent in the town and was said to have originated because that was the day when materials were collected by nailers, chain makers, locksmiths etc, and consequently little work was done. However, it became the day when the working classes enjoyed most social activities and events such as the Black Country Chartist demonstration took place (Barnsby 1980, 41).

As the population increased in Wolverhampton it soon became apparent that the religious provision in the town was insufficient (Table 3). This was not just a problem here, for nationwide the Church began to realise that the existing church accommodation in the growing towns and cities was totally inadequate. St Peter's Collegiate Church had served the people of the town since the Norman Conquest, and in 1760 the situation eased with the building of St John's in the west. But by the early 1800s this was still insufficient for the growing population so in 1834, with the help of funds from the Commissioners for Building Additional Churches, work began on St George's. The Report of the Royal Commission on Ecclesiastical Revenues of 1835 illustrates that, even after this new church was built, provision was still lacking. In addition to the Anglican churches there was a strong Nonconformist presence in the town, with Presbyterians, Unitarians, Baptists, Independents and, particularly, Methodists being represented (Robson 2002, 49–51).

Despite the apparent inadequacy of the churches to accommodate the population, there are no accurate figures of the number of people attending church, or whether they were drawn from the middle or working classes. As migration from the country to the town increased in the late 18th and early 19th centuries many people lost the habit of regular church attendance that had governed their lives in the small country villages (Chadwick 1966, 325). In addition, for some members of the working classes, the system of a pew rent based on a property qualification that operated in the town would have been prohibitive (Mander and Tildesley 1960, 165). However, the 1851 religious census, the only indicator of attendance, suggests that the average attendance on one Sunday in Wolverhampton was 53.8%, considerably higher than in nearby Birmingham with only 36.1%. The reasons for this are complex and cannot be attributed to a single factor. The cholera outbreaks in Wolverhampton produced a short-term increase in attendance, as people turned to the church for comfort when the fear of the disease was at its height, in contrast to Birmingham where the disease did not spread. Attendance at Sunday schools in Wolverhampton accounted for some of the difference and the impact of Methodism in the town was also far greater (Robson 2002, 234).

ST PETER'S COLLEGIATE CHURCH AND DEANERY
by Leonie Driver

The earliest reference to a church at Wolverhampton comes in AD 994 when Wulfrun granted land to the church here. The wording of the grant, however, implies that there was an earlier foundation and local tradition has it that the original church was founded by either by King Wulfhere of Mercia in AD 659 or King Edgar in AD 963. The church was originally dedicated to St Mary but the dedication had been changed to St Peter by the middle of the 12th century (VCH 1970, 321).

The first known charter of the church is is one of Edward the Confessor and dates from AD 1053–57. In it he pledges his troth to his priests at Wolverhampton and wills that their monastery be as free as their possessions (Mander and Tildesley 1960, 12). After the Norman Conquest William I granted the church to Samson, his chaplain and subsequently Bishop of Worcester. Samson granted the church to his cathedral priory at Worcester. The monks of Worcester lost the church of

Table 3   Church of England organisation and accommodation 1835 (Source: Robson 2002, 251)

	No. of curates	Accommodation	Population	% accommodated
St Peter	1	1,560	11,489	13.6
St John	1	1,600	6,000	26.6
St George	1	2,038	8,000	25.5

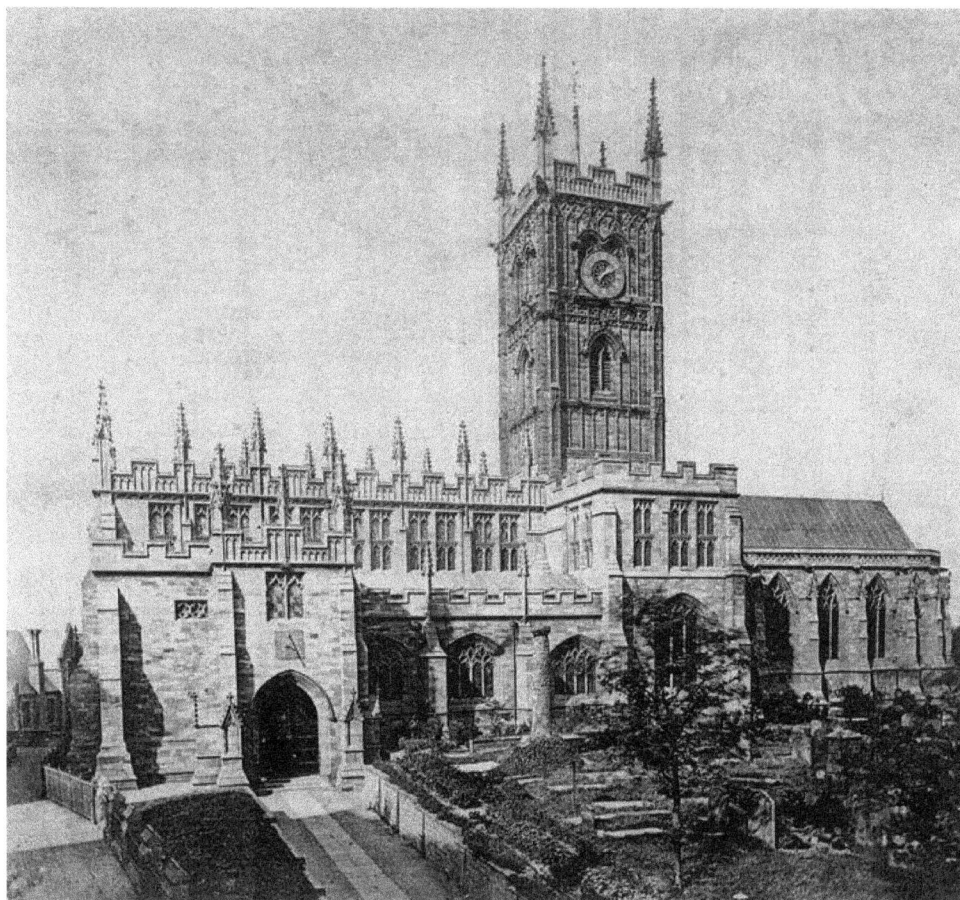

Figure 4   St Peter's Church

Wolverhampton in Stephen's reign, regained it, but then lost it again to the future Henry II in 1153–4 (VCH 1970, 322).

The church at Wolverhampton had never been a simple parish church. It was founded as a minster church from which priests would have been sent to preach in the surrounding area. In the Domesday Survey the priests of Wolverhampton are said to hold land from Sansom. By the later medieval period the church had developed into a royal free chapel with a collegiate structure of a dean and prebendaries (Slater 1986, 32).

A total of 21 deans were appointed between 1205 and *c* 1480. Few of these spent much time in Wolverhampton and the church and deanery suffered from their wastage, particularly during the 14th century (VCH 1970, 324).

The college shared the dean of St George's, Windsor, from 1457 and, following this, was annexed to Windsor in 1465 (Cockin 2000, 678). The college was dissolved for a period of three years in 1547, being restored by Mary I in 1550. The college was dissolved once again in 1645, this time being restored some 15 years later (VCH 1970, 321–31). The deanery remained annexed to Windsor until it was abolished in 1846, but the building itself was utilised for other purposes before it was demolished in 1926. The college was dissolved for the

last time in 1848 *(ibid)*. The church then became a parish church in the Diocese of Lichfield, with an incumbent entitled Rector of Wolverhampton.

The earliest parts of St Peter's Church date from the 13th century. These include the lower part of the tower and the south transept. The North Chancel, or Lanes Chancel, dates from the late 15th or early 16th century (Hall-Matthews 1993). The piers and arches of the nave are 15th century and the stone pulpit dates from 1480. The choir was fitted in 1544 with stalls taken from the dissolved monastery of Lilleshall. Parliamentary troops, quartered in the church in 1642, mutilated the interior and destroyed the records. The chancel was rebuilt in the classical style in 1682 by the dean, Dr Francis Turner. The church was extensively restored during the period 1852–65, including the addition of a new chancel, and in 1886 two new vestries were added (Cockin 2000, 678). Further restorations took place in 1937 and 1970 (Fig 4).

THE BURIAL GROUNDS *by Josephine Adams and Leonie Driver*

Burial in the land immediately around the church probably took place for many centuries and documentary evidence for this practice begins in 1539. However, this first register may be inaccurate, since it was a copy of a previous volume that had been destroyed during the Civil

War. Unfortunately, as the church was a royal free chapel, it was independent of the Diocese of Lichfield and, accordingly, unlike the situation for parish churches, there were no Bishops' Transcripts to provide a duplicate list.

St Peter's Churchyard was the only Anglican burial ground in the immediate area until 1727, when the churchyards of St Leonard's, Bilston, and St Giles', Willenhall, were consecrated. However, some people from these villages had family graves at St Peter's so they returned to bury their dead for some time.

Between 1539 and 1900, 62,031 people were listed in the St Peter's burial register. The overflow ground was consecrated in 1819 but the registers do not differentiate between the two, so it is impossible to identify which churchyard was used. Between 1750 and 1840 the numbers are inflated slightly, as some parishioners buried at St John's were listed in the register of St Peter's because their church was only a chapelry.

The number of burials recorded in the register is:

1539–1550	4
1551–1600	55
1601–1650	2,299
1651–1700	5,266
1701–1750	11,190
1751–1800	17,344
1801–1850	25,560
1851–1900	313

These figures clearly illustrate the increase in the number of burials from 1701, with the highest figure between 1801 and 1850. The number then falls dramatically as the burial ground is reaching capacity and the local cemetery opens.

The majority of burials took place in the open churchyard but there is documentary evidence in the parish burial records that lists 21 vaults along the wall on the west side of the chuchyard. This latter group is recorded with associated names and dates between 1774–97. At least two of the occupants were clergymen of St Peter's. This suggests that they may have been reserved for people of some standing in the parish. In 1841 some alterations were made to the churchyard that affected these vaults but it is not clear exactly what was done. Previously, in 1834, the controversial Dr Oliver was appointed Perpetual Curate and Sacrist of St Peters, and was said to be responsible for building an 'unsightly row of brick vaults', and reopening the old churchyard for burials. This would have been after the overflow burial ground had been opened. This was apparently unpopular with local people because it brought back memories of the cholera outbreaks of the 1830s, and by 1839 the alterations that he had made were removed (Mander and Tildesley 1960, 175).

As the number of burials increased dramatically during the 18th century, the original churchyard around the church became increasingly overcrowded. The local people were concerned, worried not only about having a place to bury their dead, but also about the unsanitory conditions that were developing. In December 1812 the *Wolverhampton Chronicle* reported that William Orgill and Joseph Smith, the churchwardens at that time, called a public meeting to discuss the necessity of establishing a new burial ground. Accompanying the advert in the December 9th 1812 edition of the *Wolverhampton Chronicle* was a letter to the editor responding to the call from the churchwardens. The letter was anonymous, but provides an invaluable account of why the establishment of a new burial ground was so necessary:

To the Editor
fari quæ sentias

SIR, – The Churchwardens having very laudably given notice of their intention to convene a meeting of the inhabitants, in the vestry of the Collegiate Church, on Friday morning next 'to consider the necessity of appointing an additional Burial Ground'. I trust you will spare me a corner in your chronicle, to state not only my own opinion, but that of many other inhabitants, that there is an immediate and pressing necessity for such an additional cemetery. And first, its necessity may be proved on the score of decency, both towards the living and the dead; for, anyone passing through the church yard, or attending the grave-digger in his daily employment, will find that he is absolutely obliged to disturb the half-decayed bodies of friends and relatives, to make even a 'narrow house' wherein to deposit those recently deceased: and farther, if you question the ancient inhabitants of this populous town, they will tell you, that in their remembrances, the ground around the church has been progressively raised by interments, to an almost incredible height above its original level. Secondly, such urgent necessity is also pointed out by a much weightier argument, viz. that of the preservation of the health of the living from the contagion of unwholesome air, which all medical men agree is a common cause of disease. For it is well known that the burying in church yards, in the midst of populous country towns, whether it arose from the effect of the increase of such towns, from ancient superstition or whatever cause, it is a bad custom; that it is habit alone which reconciles us to these things, by means of which, not only the most ridiculous, but pernicious customs, often become sacred; for certain it is, that hundreds of putrid carcasses too near the surface of the earth, cannot fail to taint the air, and that such air, when breathed into the lungs, must occasion diseases. The Jews, the Greeks, and also the Romans, well knowing this fact usually buried their dead at some distance from any town. But, Sir, I don't mean in this address to point out the precise spot where such a Burial Ground may be obtained, but to show the necessity, and importance of the parishioners fully attending the Vestry meeting, not doubting they will, after due consideration, give their support to such measures as may be deemed eligible and necessary to adopt, for the forwarding so desirable a design. – I am Sir, yours etc

AN INHABITANT

December 7th 1812

To address this problem, a Petition of Consecration, now held by the Diocese of Lichfield, details a piece of land 'one acre, one rood and twenty perches and ten square yards or thereabouts' conveyed to the incumbent on 18th June 1819. This was described as 'a parcel of land bounded on the west by a public road or way leading out of the Horsefair, on the North by land now used as a garden ground, and on the east by a Bowling Green Wall' and 'on the south by a wall and Building inclosing other land belonging to the Deanery of Wolverhampton'. This land was consecrated on 2nd October 1819. Some vaults were also built to accommodate those who, for whatever reason, did not want to be buried in the open burial ground (see Chapter 3).

On the 1750 plan of Wolverhampton by Isaac Taylor (Fig 5), that predates the establishment of the burial ground, it is not possible to locate the chosen area precisely but it was likely to include the open area behind the Deanery Hall, partly within the area of cultivated strips/ gardens, and the western part along Horse Fair, and may incorporate a few buildings situated along the western side of this road. Less detail is shown on the 1788 map by Godson; here it is also possible to see the division of fields into small plots and the area is numbered as 929.

The next large-scale map of the town of Wolverhampton was published in 1827 by Geo Wallis (Fig 5) and illustrates that the area of the development site and the part of Jennings's Gardens to the north had become 'St Peter's Burial Ground'. On the Wolverhampton Tithe map of 1842 (Fig 5) the Deanery Hall was still standing, along with several other buildings, one of which appeared to have stood within the burial ground, against its southern boundary. At this time, somewhat peculiarly, the graveyard was known as 'St Peter's New Burial Ground', some 30 years after it had been established. This may have been a distinction made between this graveyard and the original one surrounding the church itself, for the benefit of the tithe commissioners.

By 1848 this new burial ground was in turn becoming overcrowded, and again there was growing local concern about unsanitary conditions and the potential risk to health. On March 1st of that year a report of the Wolverhampton General Cemetery Company, reported in the *Wolverhampton Chronicle*, stated that 'Our graveyards are the same in extent as in 1812. Can they be suitable places at the present time? Thousands and thousands of interments have taken place, the dead lie row above row, and almost every inch is preoccupied'. The report then states that 'interments in the Old Church last year exceeded those of the preceding year by the

enormous amount of four hundred'. St Peter's had already attempted to address the problem by opening an overflow burial ground, but this too became overcrowded. The solution was to buy yet more land for another burial ground for the church that would result in an increase in local rates, or to build a cemetery paid for by the sale of shares. The newspaper article advocating the latter option was written by the Wolverhampton General Cemetery Company itself, so it may have had a vested interest! There was, however, a growing trend nationwide to favour burial in the new landscaped cemeteries that were being built, a change that could in part be attributed to a cultural change as well as practical considerations. The newly emerging middle classes, who had disposable income to spare, began to favour burial in these fashionable new cemeteries in a pleasant part of town, rather than risk the overcrowded unsanitary churchyards. A large elaborate grave memorial or family vault could signify their success in life and perpetuate their reputation in death. Subsequently, in 1849, work began on a cemetery in the town, known initially as Jeffcock Road, then Merridale Cemetery, with the first burial taking place on 12th June 1850.

After 1850 the burials recorded in the church registers fell dramatically as people began to patronise the new cemetery, and the assumption is that the majority of those listed would be in the new burial ground. However, as late as 1853 there is a record of a burial in a brick grave in the old ground, as well as interments in the vaults in both old and new grounds.

The Health of Towns map produced in 1852 is the largest scale map that shows the new burial ground. The map clearly shows the boundaries of the burial ground and the entrance to it from Horse Fair. Also shown are buildings still standing against the southern boundary of the burial ground. The gardens to the east are laid out in the same way as they appear on the map of 1750.

The First Edition O.S. map surveyed in 1889 (Fig 5) shows the burial ground almost exactly in its original form. Its boundaries appear unchanged, and there are still structures along its southern boundary. The formal gardens which occupied the area to the east have now been developed, and the site owned by Stafford Street Works, which produced tin and iron plate. The change in use of this site to industry may suggest that the burial ground was no longer in use.

The 1901 Stephens and Mackintosh Business map and the Second Edition O.S. map produced in 1902 (Fig 5) show the Deanery to be in use as a Conservative Club. The land to the northeast was owned by the School Board. An area to the south of the burial ground had been developed, and a building labelled 'Institute' has been built upon it.

Correspondence held at Staffordshire Records Office (unlisted collection D6429) illustrates that the condition

1750 Isaac Taylor plan	1827 Ged Wallis map
1842 Tithe map	1871 1871 map
1889 1st edition O.S. map	1902 2nd edition O.S. map
1919 3rd edition O.S. map	1938 O.S. map

Burial Ground   Site

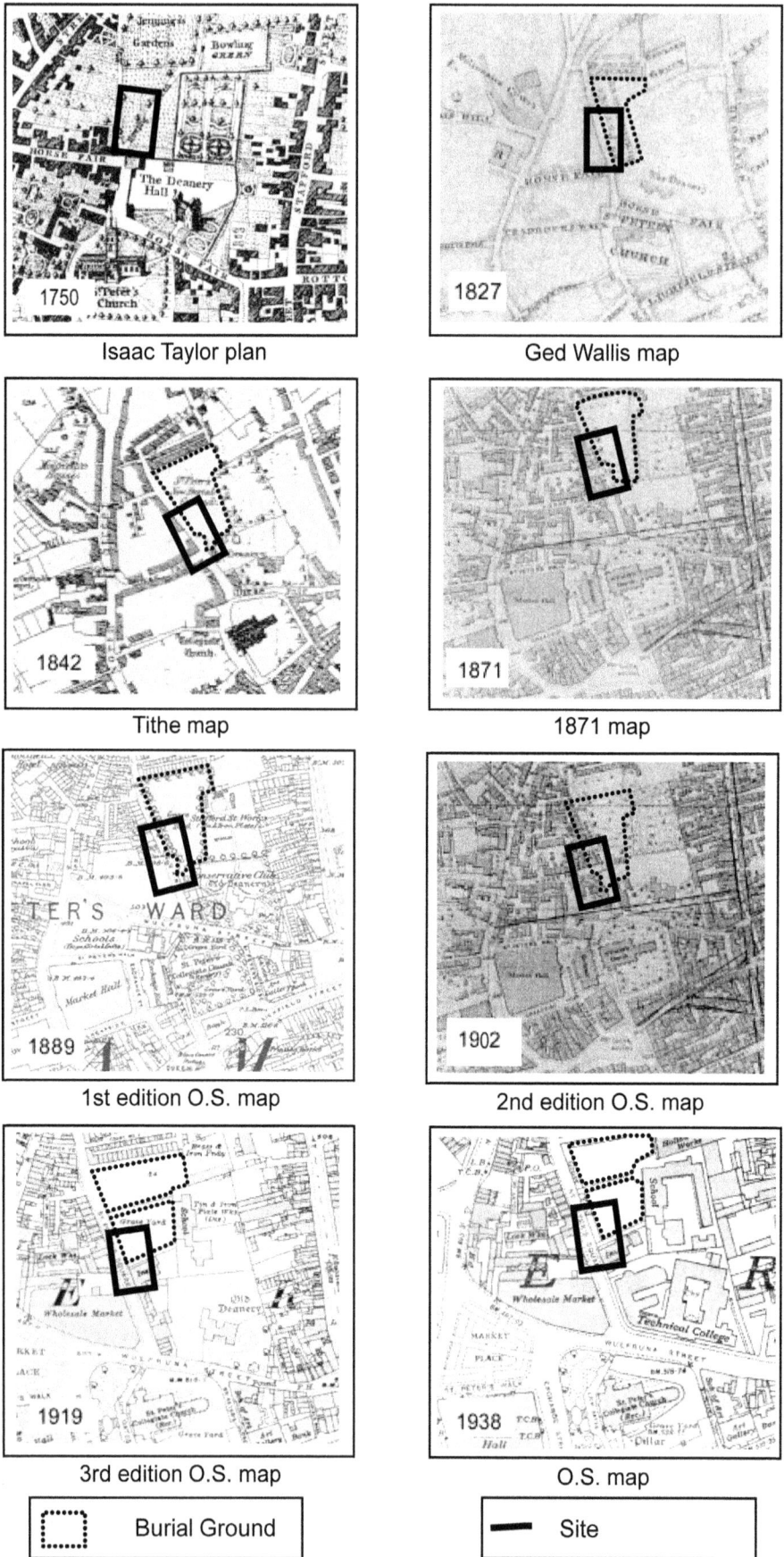

Figure 5   Selected historic maps showing location of overflow burial ground

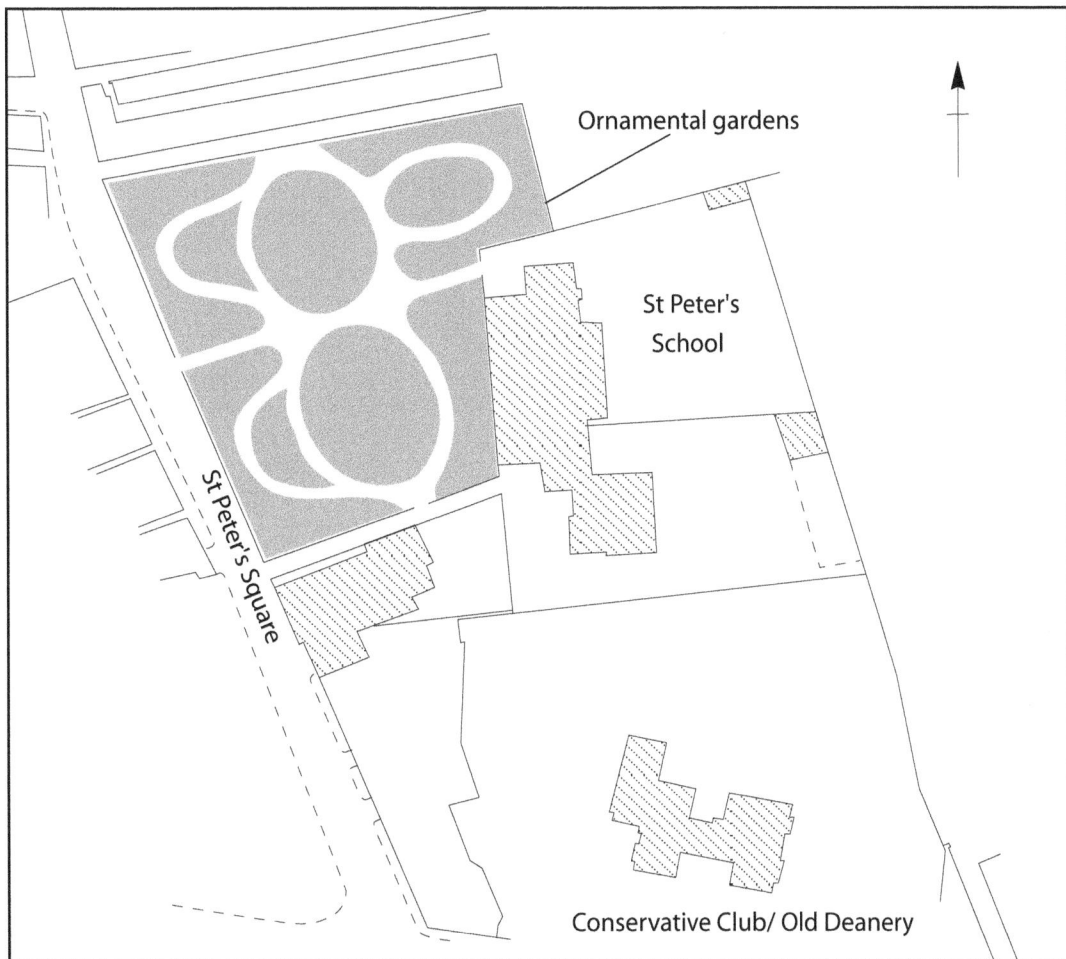

Figure 6   Plan of burial ground in 1903

of the burial ground was causing concern in 1903. The Church was faced with the choice of allowing the Town Council to make use of the land as a 'rest area', or to take on the responsibility for maintaining it themselves. A plan of the proposed changes was produced (Fig 6), but the Church decided that the cost to them was prohibitive, so agreed that the Town Council should assume responsibility for the burial ground on the understanding that 'the tombstones be reverently treated and so placed that they would not be subjected to rough usage'. It is not known however, if these alterations were actually carried out.

On the Third Edition O.S. map of 1919 the 'Grave Yard', as it is called, is still marked but now with two paths across it (Fig 5). One large one led to a school on the site of the disused plate works, while the second led to the recently constructed Institute. In 1923 the fate of the burial ground was again under discussion when the Church objected to the Council's plan to convert the area to a children's playground. However, their objection was overruled and in 1924 the plan went ahead (*ibid*,

Staffordshire RO). The Deanery was demolished in 1926 and the site was developed as a Technical College by the time of the publication of the 1938 O.S. map (Fig 5). This map also shows the widening of the central path through the graveyard and the possible development of paths around its perimeter. The school to the east is also significantly enlarged.

Subsequently, in 1973, parts of the burial ground were supposedly cleared prior to extension work to Wolverhampton Polytechnic, although no records relating to this have been found.

The church at Wolverhampton has been a focal point for the settlement for over 1000 years providing worship and ministry and a place of burial for its inhabitants. The church still dominates the centre of the city and the churchyard immediately around the church is now a garden where people can sit and rest. The overflow burial ground was finally cleared in 2001 for the construction of the Harrison Learning Centre, part of the University of Wolverhampton.

CHAPTER 3

The Archaeology

Kevin Colls and Charlotte Nielsen

EXCAVATION RESULTS

Activity on the site can be broadly divided into three phases (Neilson and Coates 2002):

Phase 1   Pre-19th-century, possible medieval, features which predate the burial ground.
Phase 2   The 19th century burial ground, including earth-cut burials and vaults.
Phase 3   Post burial ground activity, 1870 onwards.

Phase 1 (Fig 7)

Archaeological features and deposits predating the burial ground proved somewhat scarce. The earliest activity encountered on site consisted of features F214, F215 and F216. A shallow terminating gully F214 was located in the southern part of the site on a north-south alignment. Truncated to the north, the gully was cut by posthole F215 before terminating close to pit F216. The fill of F214 (1397) produced one sherd of medieval pottery dated to the mid-13th to 14th century. A further sherd of 14th- to 15th-century date was recovered from fill 1399 of pit F216.

These features predate the burial ground, but their function and wider context is difficult to determine. It is likely that the site saw medieval activity, but the later burial ground and subsequent construction has probably destroyed much of the earlier archaeology. The features and the associated artefacts still have value, as medieval deposits are rarely found in Wolverhampton. They are likely to have lain within the medieval Deanery but their function is uncertain.

Phase 2 (Fig 8)

Earth-cut burials

The earth-cut burials were concentrated in the southern part of the site. These represent just a small portion of the population of the entire burial ground as the clearance in 1973 appears to have removed earth-cut and vault burials from the north. Many of the burials encountered during excavations had been damaged by modern building activity, although the recovered assemblage was generally in good condition. The burials were broadly supine, and in most cases the position of the skeletal remains seemed to be consistent with the natural decay process. As is customary, the graves were aligned east-

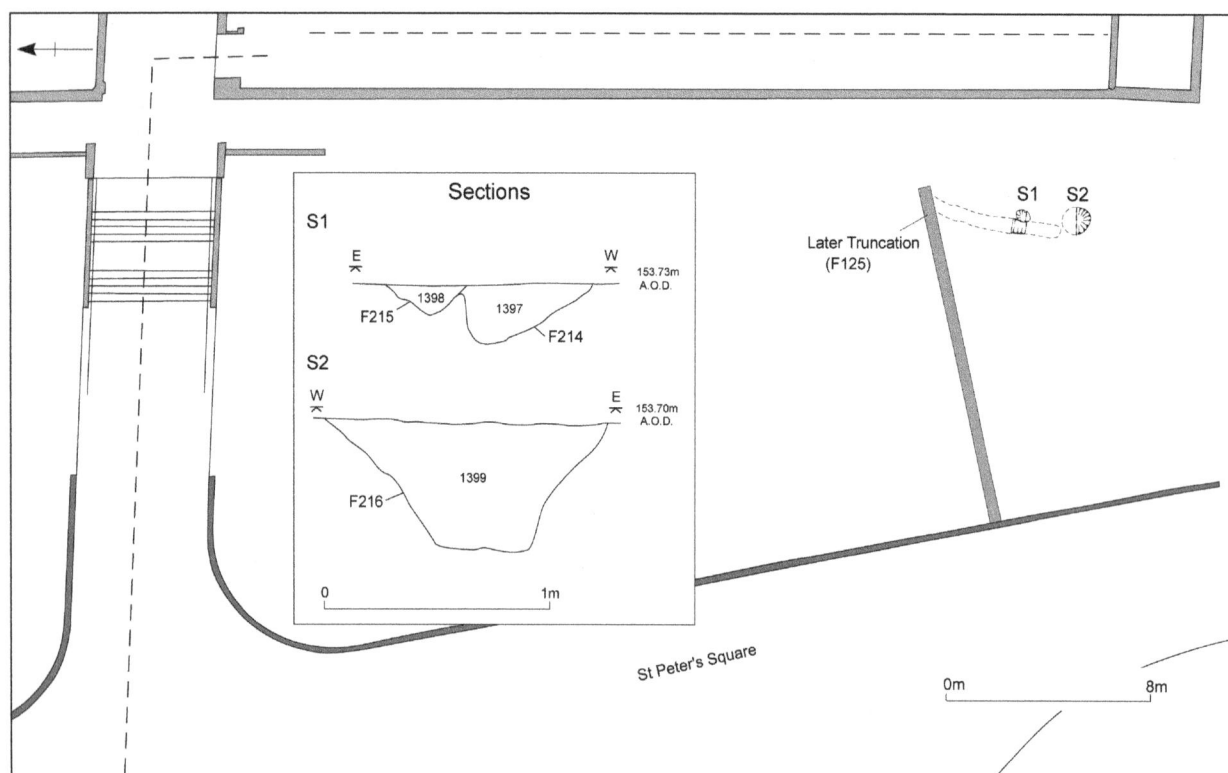

Figure 7   Phase 1 plan showing archaeological features

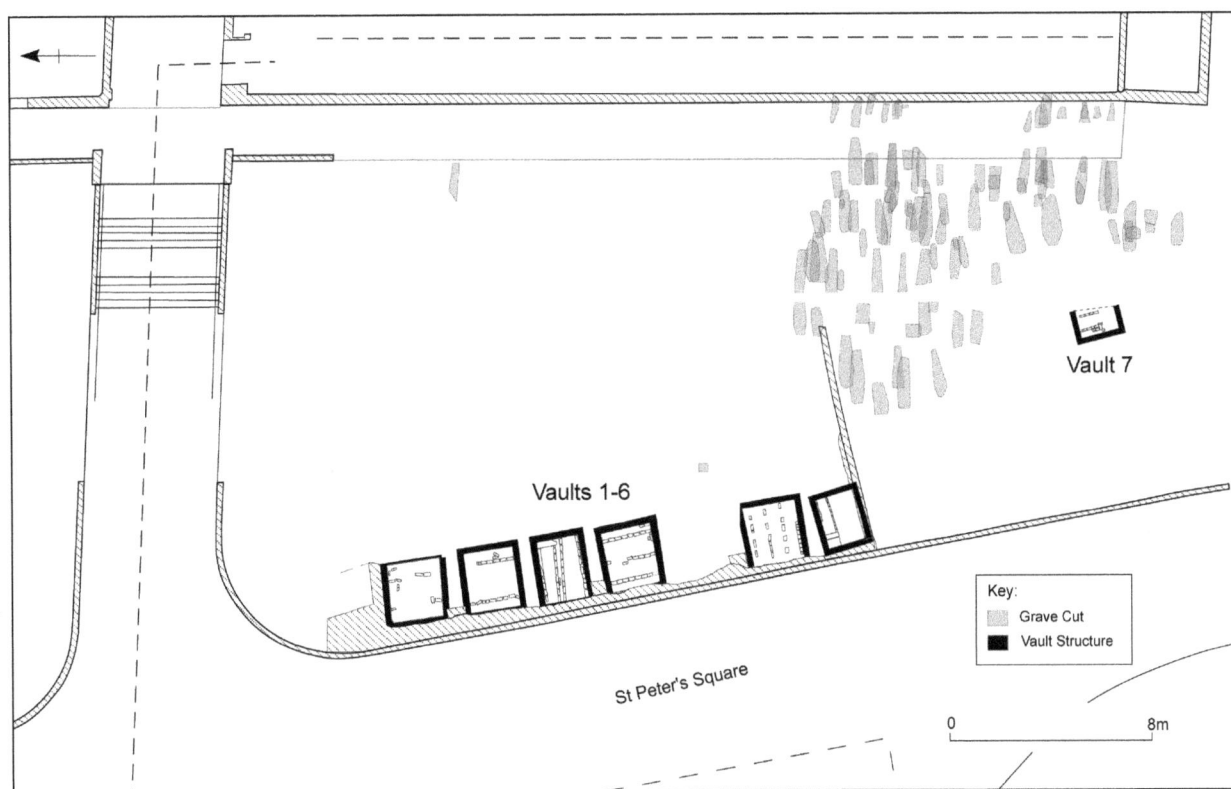

Figure 8   Phase 2 plan showing burials and vaults

west with the head at the western end (Cox 1998), with the only exception being foetal burial HB 45. Here the head was found at the eastern end, which in itself is not surprising for such a small burial.

A total of 152 burials were recorded archaeologically (Arabaolaza, Ponce and Boyston 2005; Table 4), although after skeletal analysis it emerged that, in three cases, bones of a second individual were identified amongst those of the first. These were assigned the same human burial number as the burial first identified with an additional letter added (eg 12a and 12b). Anthropological analysis was carried out on 150 articulated skeletons, of which 58 were infants and 92 were adults. Detailed analysis of preservation, sex, demography, and pathology can be found in Chapter 5.

The human skeletal remains revealed a rich and broad variety of pathological conditions such as trauma, congenital and developmental anomalies, specific and non-specific infections, metabolic diseases, neoplastic conditions, and joint related diseases. Diseases such as rickets, scurvy and *cribra orbitalia* were frequent. Three skeletons had undergone amputations (HB 53, 86, and 129), all of which were well healed. One individual demonstrated evidence of tuberculosis (HB 40) with two showing signs of syphilis (HB 44 and 75). Three skeletons produced evidence for malignant tumours (HB 39, 40 and 84), with HB 39, in particular, showing signs of a well-preserved sunburst appearance on some vertebrae and ribs. Even though it was a dramatic case

and its cause is unknown, it is possible to label it as an osteosarcoma (see Chapter 5).

The burials had been densely interred and, on occasion, there was more than one body in a grave (Plate 5). Six burials were encountered where a young individual had seemingly been buried with an adult (Table 5). Two graves, F116 and F218, were encountered each containing the remains of two adults and one juvenile or infant. Three graves, F110, F126 and F166, contained the remains of two infants in each. A further eight of the recorded graves contained the remains of two adults.

The possibility that individuals sharing grave cuts were related is difficult to assess, although there is a greater chance when individuals were recorded as sharing a single coffin. As Table 5 shows, the only two shared coffins identified both had the skeletal remains of an adult female and a juvenile (graves F122 and F191). It is possible that children were buried with adults to ease the cost of burial or to maximise space in the graveyard. Wealthier families tended to have their children buried with adult members of the family (Harding 1998). In some cases it is possible that burials containing adult and neonate remains may indicate death during childbirth. The interred remains in grave F199 were particularly intriguing, with an adult male (age 18–25) seeming to have shared the grave with an unborn fetus (estimated at 3 weeks). However, as sex determination from skeletal remains can never be certain, it is possible that the sex of the adult was misassigned.

Table 4 Human burial summary table (Source: Arabaolaza, Ponce and Boylston 2005)

Burial No.	Sex	Age (years)	Completeness (%)	Type / location	Notes
HB 1	In	18+ years	0-25%	V 4	-
HB 2	F	36-45	0-25	V 4	Osteoarthritis of thoracic spine. Deltoid enthesopathies on both clavicles
HB 3	F	18+	0-25	V 4	-
HB 4	In	18+	0-25	V 1	-
HB 5	In	36-45	0-25	V 1	Xiphoid process fused to sternal body
HB 6	In	18+	0-25	V 3	Osteoarthritis of the upper spine, new bone deposition on rib shafts, non-specific infection of both feet. Disarticulated
HB 7	In	18+	?	V 3	Disarticulated
HB 8	In	18+	?	V 2	Disarticulated
HB 9	In	18+	?	V 2	Disarticulated
HB 10	In	18+	?	V 2	Disarticulated
HB 11	In	Fet/Neo	0-25	G	Isolated burial located in the northern part of the site.
HB 12a	In	18+	0-25	V 5	Osteoarthritis of cervical spine. Cortical defect in the left superior facet joint of the axis vertebra
HB 12b	In	4-6	0-25	V 5	-
HB 13a	In	12-14	0-25	V 5	Schmorl's node on thoracic vertebra (T9)
HB 13b	In	1-4	0-25	V 5	-
HB 14	In	18+	0-25	V 5	Sacralisation of L5. Osteoarthritis of right sacro-iliac joint and costo-vertebral joints
HB 15	F	36-45	50-75	G	Osteoarthritis of lower spine T12-S1. Scoliosis and DISH
HB 16	In	1.5-2	25-50	G	-
HB 17	In	0-3 months	25-50	G	-
HB 18	In	6-12 months	0-25	G	-
HB 19	M	36-45	50-75	G	Cortical defects on right humerus
HB 20	In	8-10	75-100	G	Well preserved depositum plate found
HB 21	In	5-12 months	75-100	G	-
HB 22	M?	18-20	50-75	G	Rib lesions
HB 23	F?	26-35	0-25	G	Osteoarthritis of the right intercarpal joints, trapezio-metacarpal joints of both hands, and three hand phalanges Copper alloy ring found on finger
HB 24	In	0-2	0-25	G	-
HB 25	F?	46+	50-75	G	Osteoarthritis of cervical and thoracic spine Virtually intact china cup recovered
HB 26	In	2-3.5	75-100	G	Cribra orbitalia on both orbits. Cystic lesions above left orbit. Unusual porosity on posterior sides of both maxillae
HB 27	M?	18-20	0-25	G	Abnormal depression on right radius. Non-specific infection on right femur
HB 28	F	26-35	75-100	G	New bone formation on the visceral side of the ribs 2-10 from the left hand side
HB 29	In	1.5-2	50-75	G	-
HB 30	In	8-18 months	50-75	G	Medio-lateral bowing of right tibia and fibula
HB 31	F?	18+	25-50	G	Schmorl's nodes on upper and lower vertebral bodies of T10, T11, and L2
HB 32	M?	18+	0-25	G	New bone formation on left tibia and fibula
HB 33	M?	36-46	0-25	G	Disarticulated
HB 34	In	8-20 months	75-100	G	-
HB 35	F	36-45	50-75	G	Schmorl's nodes on T10, T12, L1 and L2
HB 36	M	46+	75	G	Osteoarthritis of the spine, right and left shoulder, left hip

Burial No.	Sex	Age (years)	Completeness (%)	Type / location	Notes
					joint, right and left hand and right foot. Non-specific infection on right tibia and fibula. Cranium with 4 osteomas. Well preserved depositum plate found lying on ribs
HB 37	F	46+	25-50	G	Osteoarthritis of the spine and the left carpo-metacarpal joint. Healed fracture on an indeterminate rib. Thickening of right rib shaft
HB 38	In	18+	0-25	G	Six healed cut marks on the cranium
HB 39	M	46+	50-75	G	Multiple perforated lesions present all over skeleton. Primary neoplasm, such as osteosarcoma. DISH on T9 to T11
HB 40	M?	36-45	25-50	G	Tuberculosis, osteochondritis dissecans on left humerus and two healed fractures on the left nasal bone and left frontozygomatic suture
HB 41	M	36-45	0-25	G	-
HB 42	F	36-45	25-50	V 7	Remains of metal ring (possible wreath) found on upper torso area. Two copper alloy rings found on the fingers
HB 43	M	36-45	25-50	G	Osteoarthritis on T8-T9-T10, severe osteophytes on L1-L2, moderate osteophytes on right clavicle, severe enthesopathies on left ulna
HB 44	M	36-45	75-100	G	Peri-mortem fractures on right femur and humerus. Syphilitic changes in right tibia
HB 45	In	Fet 33 weeks	75-100	G	Unique as head was located at eastern end
HB 46	M	36-45	75-100	G	Healed depressed fracture in the cranium
HB 47	F?	18+	25-50	G	Osteoarthritis of cervical and thoracic spine. Osteophytosis on right humerus and both calcanei
HB 48	In	6-8	75-100	G	Cribra orbitalia on left orbit
HB 49	In	1-5	0-25	G	-
HB 50	In	0-3 months	75	G	-
HB 51	F	46+	25-50	G	Osteoarthritis of the thoracic vertebrae (T5-T10)
HB 52	In	5-8 months	0-25	G	-
HB 53	F	46+	75-100	V 7	Dramatic shortening of left radius and ulna due to amputation. Disuse of left limb evident. Unusual cranial shape with exaggerated frontal bossing and crowding of dental arcade. Shroud pin found close to head.
HB 54	M	46+	75-100	V 7	Osteoarthritis of thoracic spine. Osteophytes on cervical vertebrae. Schmorl's nodes on T8, T11, and T12. Degenerative changes on both 1st ribs.
HB 55	In	9-11	75-100	G	-
HB 56	M	36-45	75-100	G	Healed oblique fracture of the left clavicle and 5th metacarpal
HB 57	M	26-35	75-100	G	-
HB 58	In	0-3 months	75-100	G	-
HB 59	F	46+	25-50	G	Non-specific infection of both humeri. Degenerative changes on the right clavicle
HB 60a	In	1-2	0-25	G	-
HB 60b	In	18+	0-25	G	-
HB 61	F	26-35	75-100	V 7	Healed fracture on the sternum
HB 62	F	46+	75-100	V 7	New bone on 10 right and left side ribs, both humeri, both scapulae, and right radius. Schmorl's nodes on T8 to T12
HB 63	In	0-3 months	0-25	G	Copper alloy button located at feet

Burial No.	Sex	Age (years)	Completeness (%)	Type / location	Notes
HB 64	In	0-3 months	50-75	G	Thickening of the skull. Non-specific infection on both scapulae
HB 65	In	6-12 months	50-75	G	-
HB 66	In	0-3 months	75-100	G	-
HB 67	F	36-45	50-75	G	Non-specific infection on left fibula. Bony formation on right tibia. Osteoarthritis of costovertebral joints. Schmorl's nodes on T11 and T12
HB 68	In	3-5	75-100	G	Cribra orbitalia on both orbits
HB 69	M	18+	0-25	G	Degenerative changes on the 11th and 12th rib heads
HB 70	M	46+	75-100	G	Medial bowing of both radii, ulnae, and fibulae. Osteoarthritis of left ulna. Congenital abnormalities of the vertebrae and ribs. Well preserved depositum plate found lying on ribs, identifying individual as James White, who died 1827 aged 42.
HB 71	In	4.5-6.5	50-75	G	-
HB 72	In	18+	0-25	V 7	-
HB 73	In	18+	0-25	NGD	-
HB 74	In	18+	0-25	G	-
HB 75	F	36-45	50-75	G	Myositis ossificans traumatica and two healed fractures on the left humerus.
HB 76	F	36-45	50-75	NGD	Osteoarthritis in vertebral column, right knee, left shoulder and right clavicle, osteochondritis dissecans on right femur
HB 77	M?	18+	0-25	G	-
HB 78	In	18+	0-25	G	-
HB 79a	In	0-1 month	50-75	G	-
HB 79b	In	0-3 months	25-50	G	-
HB 80	In	5-18 months	75-100	G	-
HB 81	M?	26-35	25-50	G	
HB 82	In	14-18	0-25	G	Cribra orbitalia on both orbits. New bone formation on both greater wings of sphenoid
HB 83	In	0-5 months	0-25	G	-
HB 84	M	36-45	50-75	G	Healed fractures of ribs, lytic lesions on ribs, vertebral bodies and os coxae - possible carcinoma? Sieve-like perforations on both humeri
HB 85	M	46+	50-75	G	Ankylosis of C2-C3 and C4-C5 possibly due to one of the seronegative spondyloarthropathies. Osteophytosis on both glenoid cavities of scapulae
HB 86	F	36-45	0-25	G	Amputation of the left tibia and fibula and osteomyelitis on the fibula, non-specific infection on both legs
HB 87	F	36-45	0-25	G	Localised new bone formation on the left tibia
HB 88	F	26-35	25-50	G	Periodontal disease, granuloma
HB 89	F	18-25	50-75	G	-
HB 90	F	46+	75-100	G	Osteoarthritis on L5 and S1. Sinusitis on left maxilla. Advanced periodontal disease
HB 91	F	18+	0-25	G	Non-specific infection on both tibiae and osteoarthritis of the right foot
HB 92	M	36-45	50-75	G	Osteoarthritis of the right elbow and L5 and S1 Healed fractures on 2 ribs. General osteophytosis
HB 93	M	18+	50-75	G	Osteoarthritis of the left shoulder, unused hip joint and right

Burial No.	Sex	Age (years)	Completeness (%)	Type / location	Notes
					temporo-mandibular joint
HB 94	In	6-12 months	25-50	G	-
HB 95	M	26-35	75-100	G	Depressed fracture located on the frontal. Localised new bone formation present on the left tibia, and both radii
HB 96	M	36-45	50-75	G	New bone on right ribs, trauma at the left 12 rib and T12
HB 97	F	26-35	50-75	G	-
HB 98	F	26-35	50-75	G	Osteoarthritis of both hands, wrist and right mid-lower thoracic rib, enthesophytes on both tibial tuberosities.
HB 99	M	36-45	50-75	G	Right external auditory meatus of the temporal bone is considerably larger than the left. Sinusitis on both maxillae
HB 100	In	6-8 months	25-50	G	New bone formation on both temporal bones
HB 101	F	16-19	50-75	G	Linear raised area on the right thoracic rib
HB 102	In	1-2	50-75	G	Antero-posterior bowing of the left femur
HB 103	In	8-15 months	75-100	G	New bone on endocranial surface of cranial vault
HB 104	F	46+	75+	G	Osteoarthritis of the cervical and lumbar vertebrae, non-specific infection on left tibia and fibula and right fibula, non-specific infection on left maxilla
HB 105	In	18+	0-25	G	Non-specific infection of both tibiae and fibulae
HB 106	In	2-3.5	75-100	G	Cribra orbitalia on both orbits. Medio-lateral bowing of both fibulae
HB 107	In	1.5-2.5	25-50	G	-
HB 108	M	18+	50-75	G	Osteoarthritis of the left acromioclavicular joint and left wrist. Degenerative changes on both first ribs
HB 109	F	46+	75	G	Osteoarthritis of the cervical spine. Healed fractures on the right ulna, 7 ribs and 5th metacarpal. New bone formation on the anterior aspect of both femora
HB 110	In	2-4	75-100	G	Cribra orbitalia on both orbits
HB 111	F	26-35	75+	G	Osteoarthritis of the right foot and left costo-manubrial joint
HB 112	M	36-45	0-25	G	Osteoma on left parietal. Osteophytosis of C3 to T6. Schmorl's nodes on T4, T7, T8, and T10
HB 113	In	3-6 months	0-25	G	-
HB 114	In	Fet	25-50	G	-
HB 115	In	18+	0-25	NGD	-
HB 116	F	26-35	75-100	G	New bone formation on the visceral side of 3 ribs. Healed fracture on the left floating rib
HB 117	M	26-35	75-100	G	Slight osteophytosis and Schmorl's nodes from T7 to T12. New bone formation on visceral side of 3 left ribs. Healed fracture of the left floating rib
HB 118	F	18-25	50-75	G	Multiple lytic lesions on both femora, humeri, radii, acromions and clavicles
HB 119	M	18-25	50-75	G	New bone formation in several areas of cranium and mandible. Cortical defects on both humeri. Schmorl's nodes on four fragments of vertebral bodies
HB 120	M	46+	75+	G	Periodontal disease, general enthesopathies, healed crushed fractures of both hands metacarpals, fracture on the nasal bone, new bone on lateral tibia
HB 121	In	15-17	25-50	G	-
HB 122a	F	46+	0-25	G	Unhealed fracture of right 10th rib.
HB 122b	F	18-25	0-25	G	-
HB 123	M?	26-35	50-75	G	-
HB 124	F?	46+	25-50	G	Osteoarthritis of the spine, two right ribs, and elbows. Myositis ossificans traumatica on right humerus. Dysplastic

Burial No.	Sex	Age (years)	Completeness (%)	Type / location	Notes
					cranium
HB 125	F?	15-18	50-75	G	Cribra orbitalia on both orbits. New bone formation on ectocranial surfaces of both greater wings of sphenoid.
HB 126	In	18+	0-25	G	Striated, lamellar, and woven bone present on the right tibia. Isolated burial located in the northern part of the site
HB 127	F	46+	50	G	Schmorl's nodes from T12 to L4.
HB 128	F	46+	50-75	G	Congenital cranio-caudal shift on one cervical vertebra. Osteoarthritis of T4 and T5.
HB 129	M	46+	50-75	G	Osteoarthritis of the acromio-clavicular joint and cervical vertebrae. Healed fracture of an unsided rib and the right femur. Amputated right femur
HB 130	M	36-45	75-100	G	Osteoarthritis of both hands and feet.
HB 131	In	13-17	0-25	G	Small hoop earring recovered and several fragments of gold plate
HB 132	In	6-12 months	50-75	G	New bone formation on a fragment from the inner table of the skull
HB 133	In	Neonate	?	G	Badly crushed. No further study
HB 134	F	36-45	50-75	G	New bone formation on the inner side of three left ribs and two right upper ribs and on the right femur
HB 135	M	46+	0-25	G	-
HB 136	In	5-7	0-25	G	Cribra orbitalia on the right orbit
HB 137	In	1.8-3.5	75-100	G	-
HB 138	F?	14-17	25-50	G	Long-standing infectious process (osteitis) on right femur. Asymmetry of the hip joints
HB 139	In	5-7	50-75	G	-
HB 140	?	adult	?	G	Not investigated. Incinerated due to mercury contamination. Well preserved depositum plate found
HB 141	In	18+	0-25	G	Schmorl's nodes on unidentifiable thoracic vertebra
HB 142	In	1.5-2	25-50	G	Cribra orbitalia on both orbits
HB 143	M	46+	0-25	G	Osteoarthritis or spondyloarthropathy of the spine. Spondylosis deformans of the cervical and upper thoracic spine. Osteoma on skull
HB 144	In	Adult	?	G	Left in situ. Partially covered by concrete
HB 145	In	Infant	?	G	Left in situ. Partially covered by concrete
HB 146	M	36-45	25-50	G	Large indentation on the left femur, Osteoarthritis of the right elbow, Schmorl's nodes and osteophytosis on the vertebrae and healed oblique fracture of a rib
HB 147	In	12-16	50	G	-
HB 148	M	18+	50	G	Osteophytosis of most joints and bone margins. Myositis ossificans traumatica on left femur
HB 149	F	46+	25-50		Spondylosis deformans on two middle thoracic vertebra and three lower thoracic vertebra
HB 150a	In	6-12 months	0-25		Abnormal remodeling and porous thickening on one left rib
HB 150b	In	5-8 months	0-25		-
HB 151	In	6-15 months	0-25		-
HB 154	In	3-6 months	0-25		-

Key: M = Male   G = Earth-cut grave
      F = Female   Neo = Neonate   V = Vault
      In = Indeterminate   Fet = Fetal   NGD = no grave defined

Table 5   Summary of graves with two or more individuals

Grave	Adult (sex) (18 years +)	Juvenile (1-12 years)	Infant (1-12 months)	Fetus/ Neonate (up 1 month)	Sequence (earliest first)	Coffin evidence
F108	HB 15 (F)	HB 16			HB 16, HB 15	No
F110			HB 17 & 18		HB 17, HB 18	No
F116	HB 27 (M), HB32 (M)	HB 24			HB 24, HB 27, 32	Coffin each
F122	HB 31 (F)	HB 29			HB 31 beneath HB 29	Shared coffin
F126			HB 34 & 80		HB 80, HB 34	Coffin for HB 080 only
F128	HB 35 (F), HB37 (F)				HB 35, HB 37	Coffin each
F131	HB 36 (M), HB46 (M)				HB 46, HB 36	Coffin each
F133	HB 39 (M), HB40 (M)				HB 39, HB 40	Coffin each
F152	HB 60b (?)	HB 60a			-	-
F166			HB 79a & HB 79b		-	-
F171	HB 85 (M), HB90 (F)				HB 90, HB 85	Coffin each
F185	HB 101 (F), HB108 (M)				HB 108, HB 101	Coffin each
F191	HB 111 (F)	HB 107			HB 111 beneath HB 107	Shared coffin
F196	HB 116 (F), HB120 (M)				HB 120, HB 116	Coffin each
F199	HB 119 (M)			HB 114	HB 119, HB 114	Coffin each
F201	HB 122a (F), HB122b (F)				?	?
F202	HB 123 (M), HB124 (F)				HB 124, HB 123	Coffin each
F218	HB 137 (?), HB 138 (F)		HB 151		HB 138, HB 137, HB151	Coffin each for adults. 151?
F222	HB 141 (?)		HB 150		HB, 141, HB 150	Coffin for 141. 150?

Although assessed for spatial distribution, there appeared to be no correlation between age at death and burial location. The evidence suggests a random distribution of burials from across the age range, regularly demonstrated by infant and juvenile burials intercutting adult burials (and *vice versa*). However, this supposition must be treated carefully as only a small part of the total area of the burial ground was excavated. The analysis, however, did demonstrate that the majority of the infants and juveniles were interred in graves far shallower than the adults, with deep child burials being infrequent.

Coffins

The preservation of the coffins was generally poor, although occasionally parts of coffins were encountered which were in good condition. Some burials were found with no identifiable coffin remains. These interments were probably in wooden coffins which have subsequently rotted away; burials in shrouds alone were not common during this period. Many of the burials were found with the decayed remains of the *depositum* plate from the front of the casket, and some still contained legible inscriptions when excavated. The best preserved *depositum* plate was from adult burial HB 70 (Plate 3). Rectangular in shape, the plate was found lying on the ribs and curving around the torso. It was black with gold-coloured lettering, which tended to fade after it had been exposed to the air. The writing on the plate read 'James Whit..., Died May 20th 1827, Aged 42 Years' (see Chapter 6).

Adult burial HB 36 also had the remnants of its *depositum* plate resting on the torso (Plate 6, and see Chapter 6). This plate read 'William Brise, Died Jan 22nd

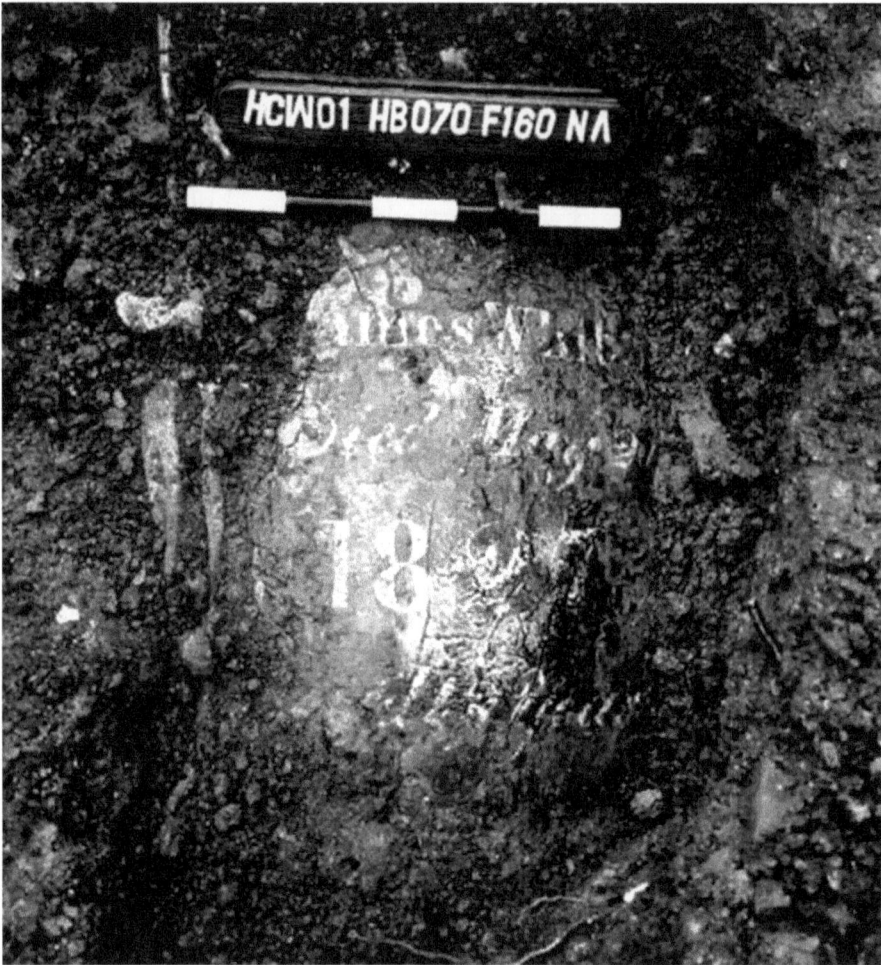

Plate 3   *Depositum* plate with HB 70

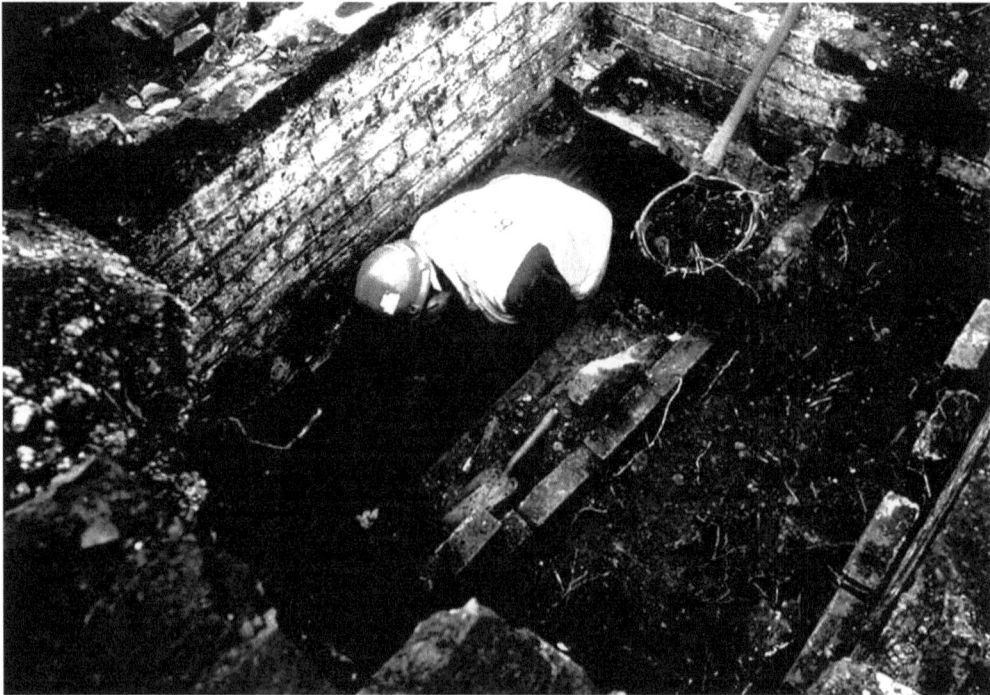

Plate 4   Excavating a vault

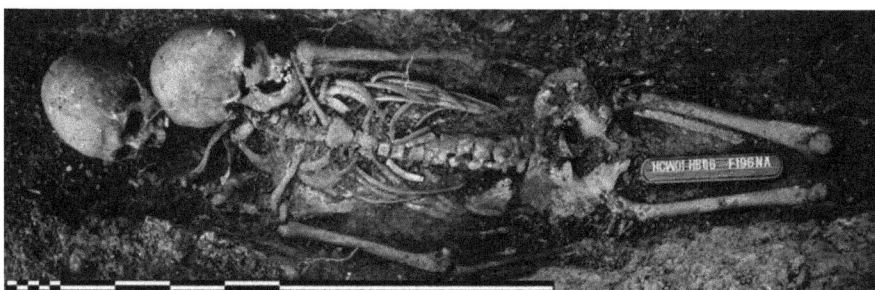

Plate 5   Two individuals interred in the same grave

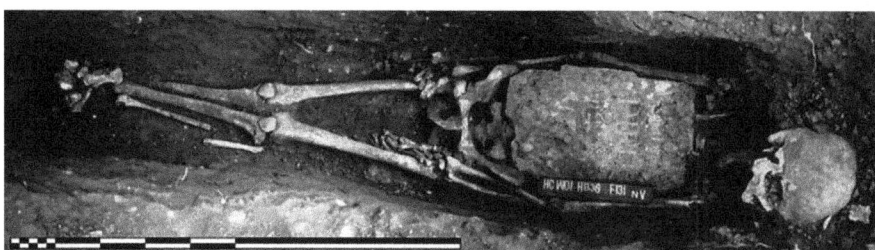

Plate 6   *Depositum* plate with HB 36

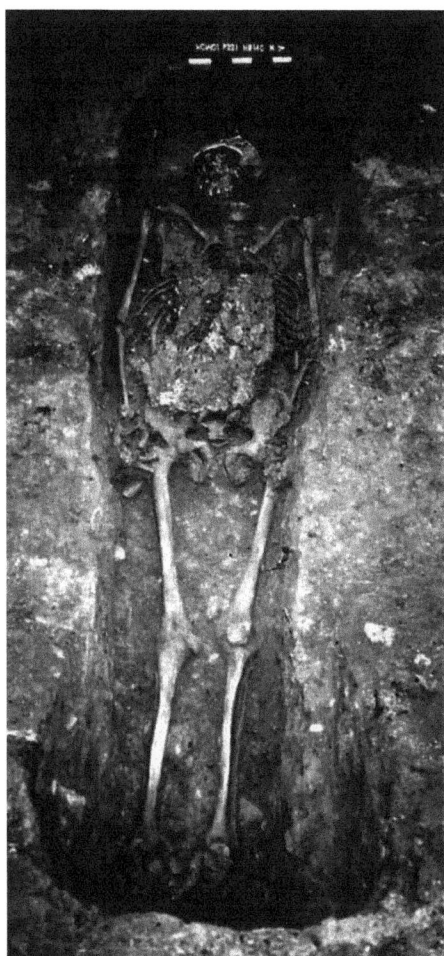

Plate 7   HB 140

18.., Aged ...'. A *depositum* plate associated with HB 20, a juvenile, had mostly decayed and the only legible word was the name 'Rachel'.

HB 140

HB 140, an adult burial, is worthy of special mention (Plate 7). During excavation, mercury was noted around the lower abdominal area of the body. The quantity of mercury was substantial enough to require treatment as contaminated waste. Subsequently the skeleton and its associated coffin material had to be incinerated and could not be taken back to the university for specialist examination. The mercury appeared to derive from within the grave and not to have seeped in from another source. A fragmentary *depositum* plate was associated with the burial. The plate still had the letters 'ayli' remaining, which could relate to the name 'Baylis' (Chapter 6).

The finds

Relatively few grave goods were found in association with the burials, which is to be expected from burials interred in a Christian tradition. Three copper alloy rings were found on the fingers of adult skeletons, one was associated with HB 23, a young middle adult possible female, and two with HB 42, an old middle adult female in Vault 7. A copper alloy button was found at the feet of a juvenile HB 63 and a small hoop earring was found with juvenile HB 131. A china cup was found with an adult burial, HB 25, and was virtually intact with only the handle missing.

The vaults (Fig 9)

Seven vaults were encountered on the site and all were excavated individually (Plate 4). Vaults 1 to 6 were

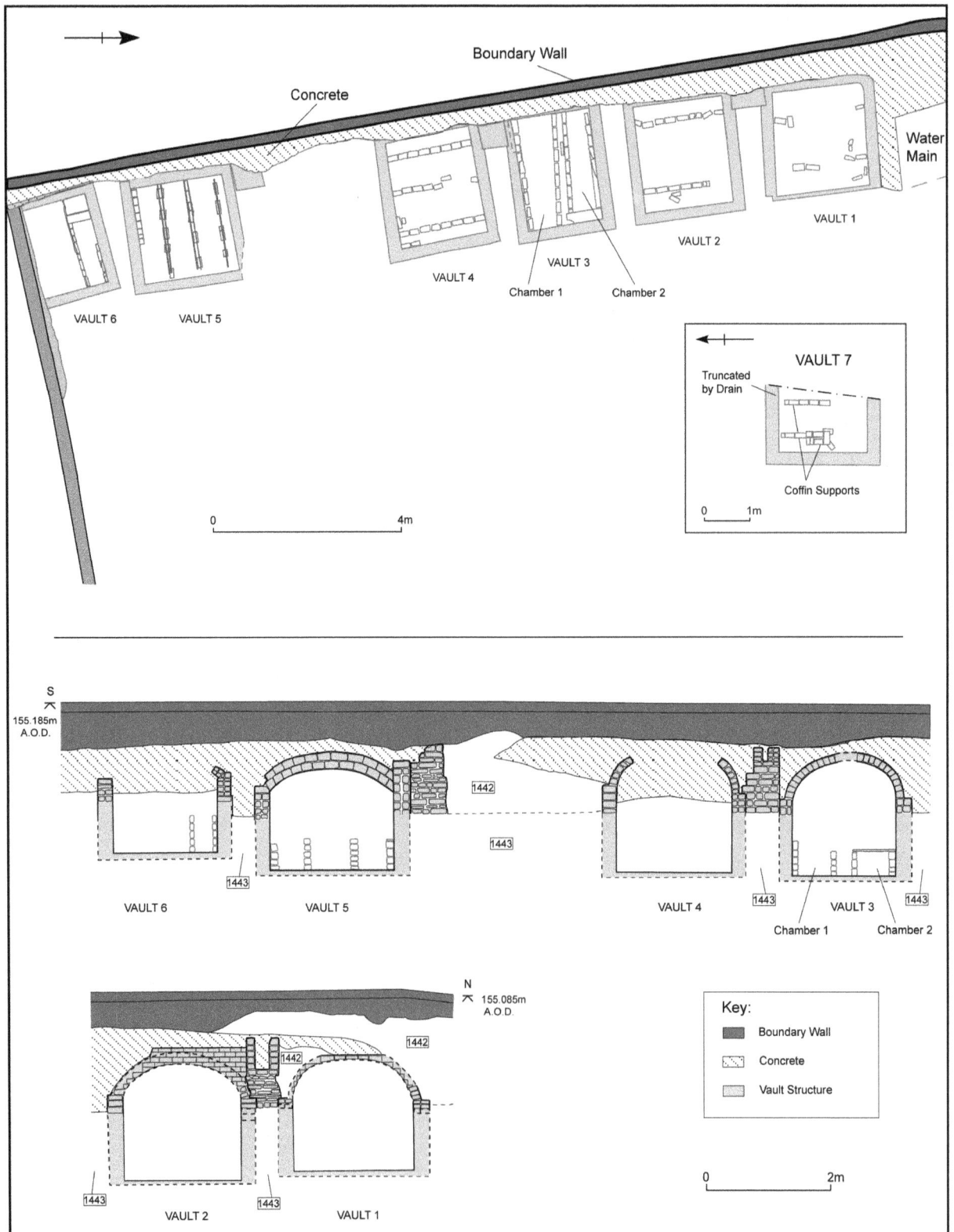

Figure 9   Phase 2 profile of the vaults

located along the western boundary of the site, with Vault 7 encountered further to the south. All were similar in style and character and were constructed in the 19th century when the graveyard was in use. Although the remains of only seven vaults were encountered, it seems likely that more were present prior to the site clearance in 1973. Vaults 1 to 6 appear to have been subject to clearance, leaving mostly intact walls but no complete roofs. They were filled with a mixture of modern rubble and debris. Vault 7 was found to be intact. All were constructed of machine-cut red bricks and were orientated east-west (see Table 6).

Table 6 Vault summary table

Vault number	External dimensions	Roof	Floor	Internal divisions/features	Human burials
1	2.24m x 1.96m	Barrel vaulted roof, destroyed	Brick	No divisions. Interior white washed. Padlocks and coffin supports present	HB 4 and 5
2	2.50m x 2.42m	Barrel vaulted roof, destroyed	Brick	Interior whitewashed with coffin supports present	HB 8,9 and 10
3	1.89m x 1.68m	Barrel vaulted roof, destroyed	Brick, herringbone pattern	Two chambers, divided by brick walls with void, sealed by sandstone slabs	HB 6 and 7
4	2.17m x 1.85m	Barrel vaulted roof, destroyed	Brick	Interior whitewashed with coffin supports present	HB 1, 2 and 3
5	2.46m x 2.45m	Barrel vaulted roof, mostly destroyed	Brick	Three chambers, sealed by slabs. Divisions consisting of brick, slabs and metal bars. Whitewashed	HB 12a/b, 13a/b, and 14
6	2.63m x 2.07m	Barrel vaulted roof, mostly intact	Brick	Two chambers, sealed by slabs. Mostly destroyed. Whitewashed	Disarticulated human remains
7	2.30m x >1.55m	Barrel vaulted roof, collapsed	Brick	No divisions. Brick coffin supports, iron bracket. Plastered	HB 42, 53, 54, 61, 62, and 72

Vault 1

Vault 1 was the northernmost vault of the six and was constructed of machine-cut, red bricks with lime-washed internal walls. The profile of the roof and some of its remains could be seen in section against the wall on the western boundary of the site. The vault measured 1.84m from the floor to the apex of the roof. The vault had a barrel-vaulted roof, most of which had probably been destroyed during the clearance. The floor of the vault was bordered by a series of half bricks and the floor itself consisted of east-west aligned stretchers. Two disturbed rows of unmortared brick coffin supports were found, one at the east end of the vault and one at the west end.

Only the partial remains of two skeletons (HB 4 and 5) and two coffins were found in the vault. It is impossible to say exactly how many bodies were originally in this vault. It is likely that the remains found had been missed during the clearance or had fallen out of the decomposed coffins when they were lifted. One fragment of grave memorial, found within the fill of the vault, had the name 'Collins' inscribed on it (Chapter 6). It is possible that this name relates to one of the bodies located within this vault, but it is also possible that this grave memorial was simply thrown in with the backfill during the clearance and could have originated from anywhere in the burial ground.

Vault 2

Vault 2 was very similar to Vault 1, a rectangular brick-built vault with evidence to demonstrate a barrel-vaulted roof prior to destruction (Plate 8). The entry to this vault seemed to be in the southeast corner of the east-facing wall. The ninth course of bricks was laid as headers and the entry point was immediately on top of this. This corresponded to the level of the ground surface into which the vault was cut. The floor of the vault consisted of stretchers, aligned in roughly east-west rows, and was laid directly on to natural sandstone.

This vault was linked to Vault 1, at the western end, by a narrow brick wall between the two vaults (Plate 8). Vault 2 also had remaining evidence of two coffin supports, which were disrupted but aligned north-south. This vault had also been cleared, although the disarticulated remains of three skeletons (HB 8, 9, and 10) were found in the vault fill. The only remaining evidence of coffins was several coffin handles, which were all corroded and not found *in situ*. Two fragments of grave memorials were found within the fill of Vault 2. Only one piece had a name on it, but it was incomplete and may not have derived from this vault.

Vault 3

Vault 3 was similar in design and build to the other vaults (Plate 9). The entry to this vault was also at the east end, possibly at the top of the ninth course of bricks. The vault had two internal chambers constructed of unmortared red bricks, which were not bonded to the build of the main vault. The style of each chamber suggested that they were constructed at different times and possibly by different people. The north wall of Chamber 1 was not straight and aligned slightly to the southeast; this was probably done to accommodate the shape of the coffins. Between the two chambers was a small void, and each chamber had originally been sealed with sandstone slabs. The floor of the vault was made of bricks laid in a herringbone pattern. This was the only vault with this floor pattern.

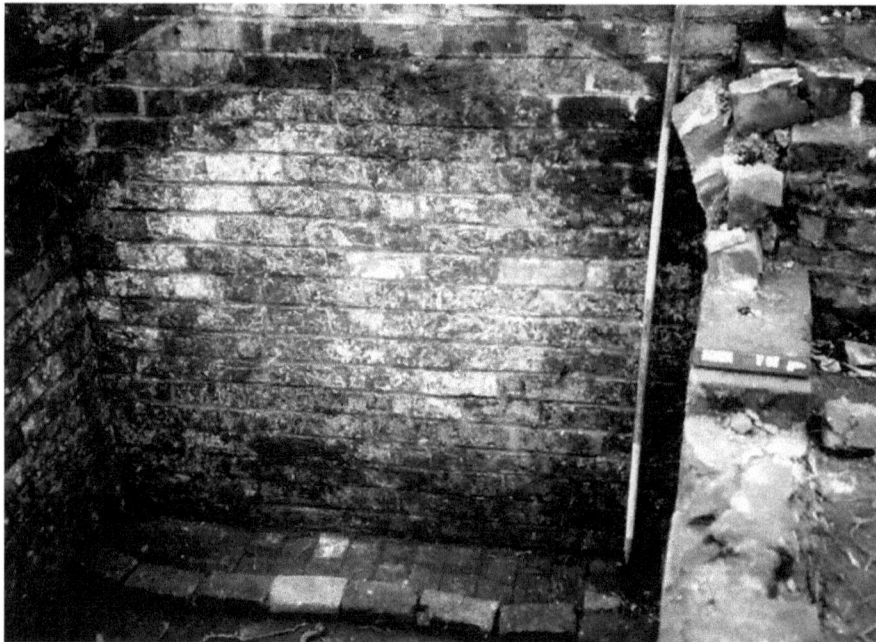

Plate 8   Vault 2

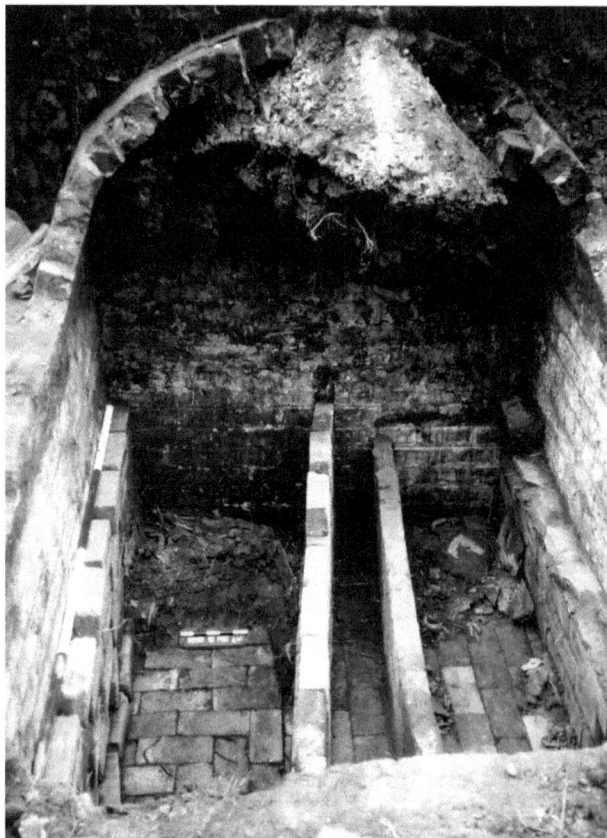

Plate 9   Vault 3

In situ coffin remains were identified in each chamber. Although both coffins had decomposed, or had been removed during the clearance, much of the western end (head end) of both coffins remained. No articulated bones were found in conjunction with these coffins, but clusters of disarticulated bone, mainly the bones of the hands and feet, remained approximately *in situ*. These represented two bodies (HB 6 and 7). It is probable that the remainder of the remains had been removed during the 1973 clearance. If the coffins had been badly preserved at the time of the clearance then it is possible that some remains of coffins and bones were left behind. It is also possible that more bodies existed within the vault, placed on the sandstone slabs. No grave memorials with discernible names were found within the fill of this vault.

Vault 4

Vault 4 was rectangular in plan and constructed from machine-cut red bricks. The roof was barrel vaulted, although mostly destroyed. The floor of the vault was made of unmortared bricks, laid in rows, aligned approximately north-south and laid directly onto the natural sandstone. Placed on the floor were three unmortared coffin supports. They each consisted of a single line of bricks, aligned north-south. The middle row of bricks had been slightly disturbed.

Some disarticulated bones were found within the fill of the vault, lying on the floor. These were only scant remains, as the majority of the bones were probably removed during the clearance of the burial ground. The bones were found in clusters and represent the partial remains of three individuals (HB 1, 2, and 3).

The fill of Vault 4 produced five fragments of the same grave memorial. The only writing on these pieces consisted of a name: 'T. Ford' (Chapter 6). It is possible that this sandstone memorial relates to one of the occupants of this vault but, again, the disturbance caused by the clearance meant that this memorial could have been deposited with the backfill and may be from another part of the site.

Vault 5

Vault 5 was again similar in construction to the other vaults. The preservation of the roof of this vault was slightly better as not all the roof had been destroyed. At the eastern end of the vault, the roof was partially intact and made of a single skin of bricks. The vault had been backfilled with modern rubble and soil. When this was removed a layer of slabs was revealed. The slabs would

have acted as a seal on the bottom layer of coffins and provided another level on which to place coffins. Most of this layer had collapsed, with only the northern part surviving *in situ*. The slabs were supported by three rows of red brick supports creating three chambers within the vault (Plate 10).

The remains of five individuals (HB 12a/b, 13a/b, and 14) were identified within the vault. Two were the remains of young adults, two were children, and one was an infant (Table 4). The skeletal remains were recovered from the three lower chambers in the vault along with the remains of three decomposed wooden coffins. Seven fragments of grave memorials were recovered from the fill of Vault 5, only one of which was of any significant value. This was a gravestone, which although broken off at the centre carried a full inscription. The inscription related to a Thomas Fullwood, who died in 1864, his wife Mary, who died in 1860 and their son, Thomas, who also died in 1860 aged 34 years (Chapter 6). It is possible that this was the grave marker for Vault 5 and that the bones found within it belonged to the children of Thomas and Mary. However, this stone may have originated elsewhere and merely been deposited with the backfill. One other grave memorial fragment from this vault had the name 'Samuel' on it, but no other relevant information regarding the person could be established.

Vault 6

Vault 6 was the southernmost vault in the row and was also rectangular in plan with a barrel-vaulted roof. Vault 6 was different to Vaults 1 to 5 in that the roof was virtually intact. However, the eastern wall of the vault and part of the roof at the eastern end had been destroyed, presumably to aid the 1973 clearance. The vault was also on a slightly different alignment to the other vaults, being positioned northeast to southwest. The interior of the vault had been lime washed and the vault had a brick floor laid directly on to the natural sandstone.

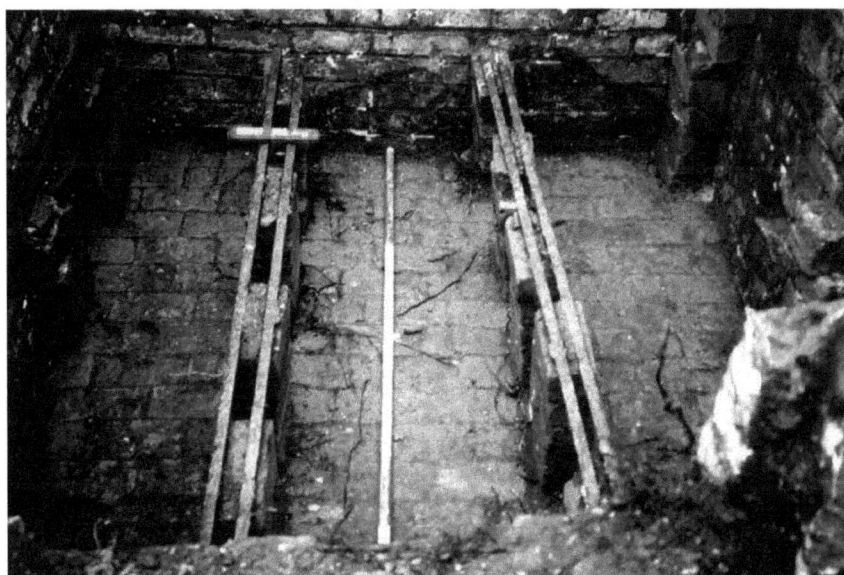

Plate 10 Vault 5

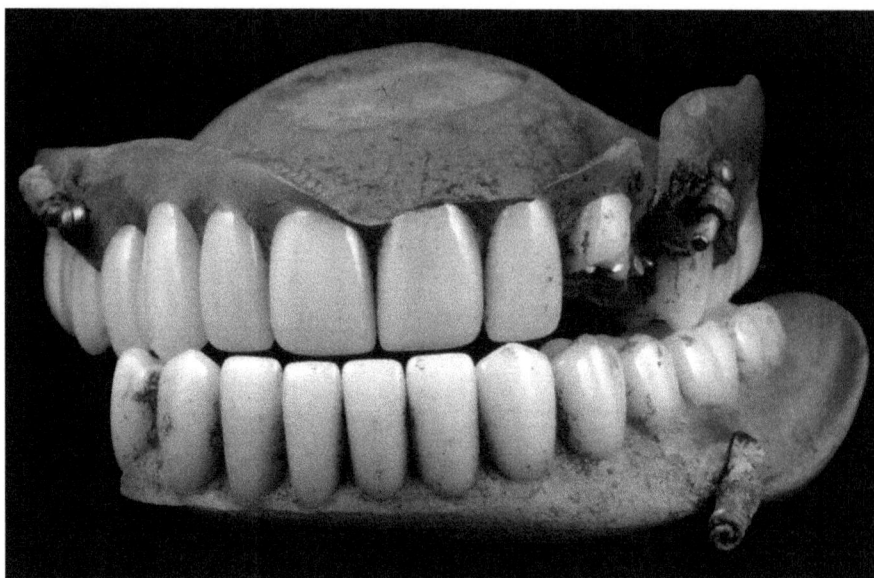

Plate 11 Dentures from Vault 6

Vault 6 had been divided into two chambers by a single row of bricks, curved to fit round the shape of a coffin. The northern chamber was much narrower than the southern one. Two drystone sandstone slabs covered the western end of the narrow chamber. Originally other slabs may have sealed both chambers, allowing further coffins to be placed on top, but no evidence survived. It is possible that the narrow chamber was designated for a juvenile, although it is difficult to prove this as only disarticulated bones were recovered from the fill of the vault. The coffin material and bones from this vault had been considerably disturbed so it was not possible to determine the exact number of skeletons or coffins that were present. Also found in the fill of Vault 6 were a set of vulcanite dentures (Plate 11, and see Chapter 4).

A cracked, but complete, grave memorial stone was found in the fill of Vault 6, which may or may not relate to the occupants of the vault. The inscription has the names of three people from the same family on it: John Carter who died in 1864, his wife Mary who died in 1877, and their son Thomas Watwood Carter who died in 1871 aged 15 years. This stone also had an unusual feature as it had an image of a skeleton carved over the inscription (Plate 12). This appeared to be a modern graffito and not the work of the original stonemason. This suggests two possibilities. Either the grave memorial was defaced as it stood marking the occupants of this vault prior to 1973, and was placed in the vault during the clearance, or the memorial was defaced during the clearance, in which case it may have originated from elsewhere and not relate to this vault at all.

Vault 7

Vault 7 was not situated in the same row as Vaults 1 to 6, but to the southeast (Fig 8). It was similar to the other vaults in character, but was better preserved, although truncated by a modern storm drain. The roof of Vault 7

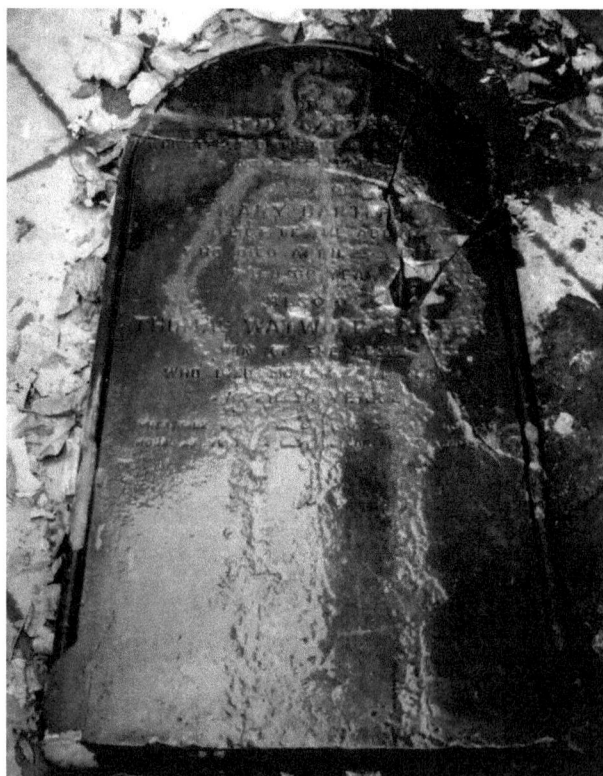

Plate 12 Graffiti on headstone of Thomas Carter, Vault 6

had collapsed, but appeared to have been a barrel-vaulted roof, with some of the upper courses of brick missing. This vault had not been cleared in 1973.

Internally, the walls had been plastered with a light grey mortar and an iron bracket was still attached to the wall in the southwestern corner (Plate 13). A similar iron bracket, with wood still attached, was found in the fill of Vault 7, which suggests that these brackets may have been used to support small coffins. The brick floor of the

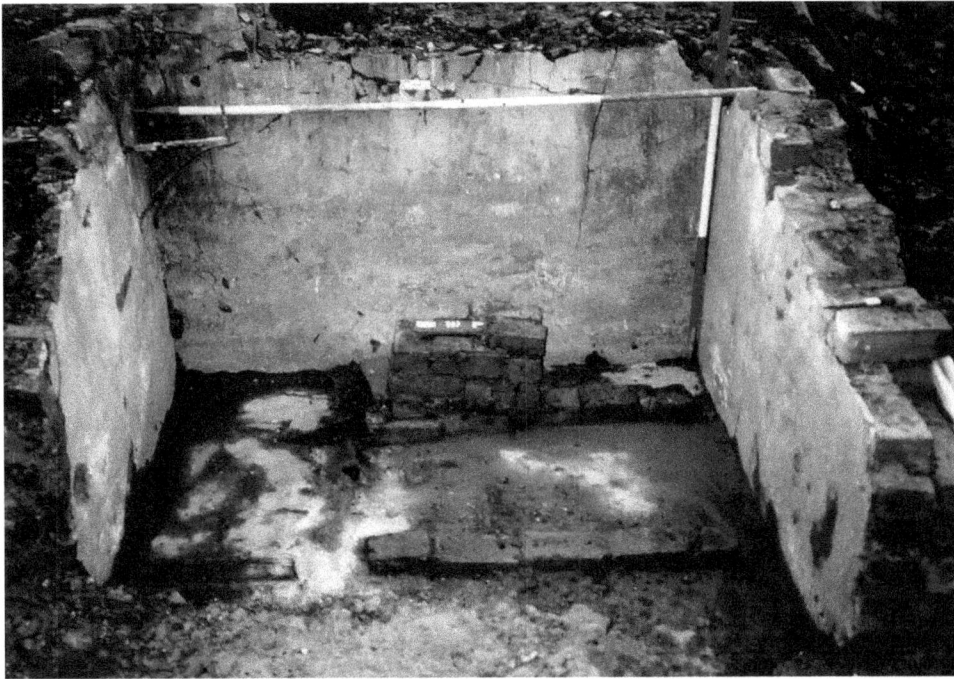

Plate 13 Vault 7

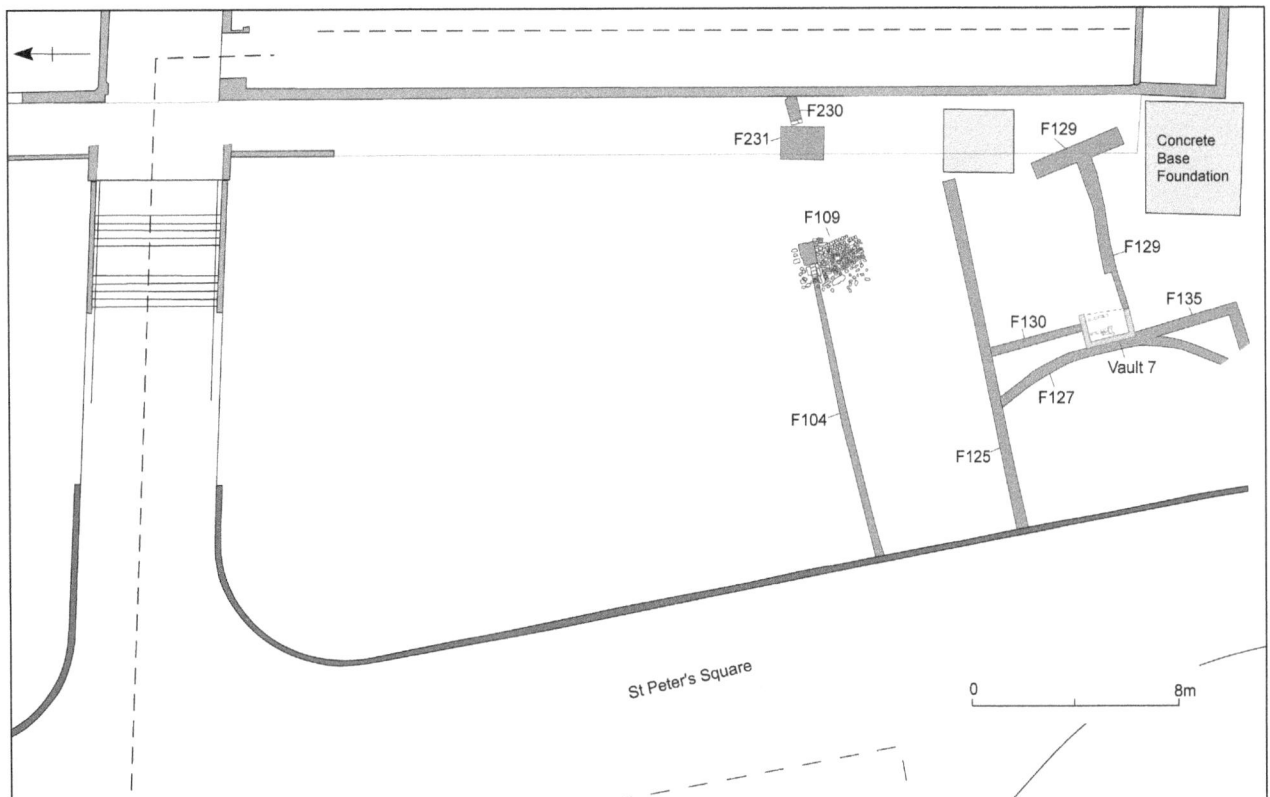

Figure 10 Phase 3 plan showing post-burial ground activity

vault was laid directly onto the natural sandstone. The bricks were laid in rows, aligned approximately north-south. Two brick coffin supports were found in the northern part of the vault; these supports were mortared to the brick floor.

Six adult skeletons (HB 42, 53, 54, 61, 62 and 72) were recovered from this vault. The top layer of remains was from HB 53, HB 42 and HB 61; underneath were HB 54, HB 72 and HB 62 respectively. Originally, the coffins would have been stacked on top of each other but during the decompositional process the bodies and coffins in the top layer had collapsed onto the lower coffins. The skeletons were mostly intact, except where the storm drain had truncated the vault and had destroyed the skeletons below the knees. In the fill near to the head of HB 53 a shroud pin and lead fragments were found with the wooden coffin remains. These fragments may have originated from a *depositum* plate, or may have been the remains of a lead-lined coffin. This was difficult to determine as the coffin had mostly decomposed.

On the chest of HB 42 were the remains of a metal ring, which may have been the remains of a wreath placed on the coffin. Floral tributes did not become fashionable until the 1860s (Litten 1991), which corresponds with the possible dates of the later burials within the family vaults.

A copper alloy ring was also found on the finger of HB 42. Evidence of *depositum* plates was found with the skeletons in Vault 7, but they were in such a poor state of preservation that they were illegible. No grave memorials were found in association with this vault, so it was not possible to establish the identities of any of the human remains within the vault.

A later wall (F127, Fig 10) had been incorporated into the build of the southern wall of Vault 7. The curvilinear brick wall, four courses in height, may represent the remains of the southwestern boundary wall of the burial ground as shown on the 1842 tithe map and again on the plan of Wolverhampton dated 1871 (Fig 5). No burials were truncated by, or were identified to the east of, wall F127.

Phase 3
During the excavations a series of 20th-century walls and a brick surface were identified (Fig 10). Located at the southern end of the site, these features closely match the location of St Peter's School, built in the early 20th century (Fig 5). Constructed from machine-cut red bricks sitting on concrete foundations, the walls often truncated burials. However, burials located between these later structures were generally unaffected. Walls F125, F129, F130, and F135 probably represent the partial footprint of St Peter's School. Wall F104 (and continuation F230) closely corresponds to the location of the new southern boundary wall of the burial ground constructed in association with St Peter's School during the early 20th century (Fig 5).

CHAPTER 4

The Finds

SMALL FINDS
by Lynne Bevan

The small finds consisted of three copper alloy finger rings, part of a gold earring and some small gold fragments, a halfpenny, part of a button or stud and a rectangular piece of worked bone, possibly a handle.

The rings were in a very poor state of preservation. Two of the rings came from the grave containing HB 42, a middle adult female in Vault 7. The wider of the two rings appears to have been plain, although any decoration might have been obscured by surface degradation, and the bezel of the other ring, which is broken, was originally inlaid with five stones, only two of which remained *in situ*. The appearance of the two remaining stones was cloudy and opaque, suggesting that they might be made of glass. The third ring found with HB 23, a middle adult, probably female, in an earth-cut grave, might have had a decorated surface but this remains uncertain due to its poor condition. All the rings were small and appear to have belonged to females.

The small hoop earring was discovered with HB 131, an adolescent burial in an earth-cut grave. Only half was present, and although plain, it was well preserved. A few small fragments of gold plate, one of which was circular, came from the same burial. These might relate to the earring, or another small item in the burial. Part of a copper alloy button or stud was recovered from burial HB 63, an infant burial in an earth-cut grave. This consisted of a curved, circular disc with an attachment loop, which was probably from a dress coat. It is unlikely, therefore, that the button was directly associated with the burial. A 19th-century date is probable for this item.

The coin was recovered from the fill of Vault 6. Although in a very poor state of preservation, it has been identified as a George III halfpenny dating to the 1790s or the early 19th century.

A polished bone object was recovered from the grave containing HB 101, an adolescent or young adult female in an earth-cut grave. The surface appears worn, and was probably used as a handle. While it was too narrow to have hafted a knife it could have been attached to another implement. Such undiagnostic fragments are not generally datable.

A metal ring found on the chest of HB 42 may have been the remains of a wreath placed on the coffin.

POTTERY
by Stephanie Rátkai

All the pottery was examined macroscopically and divided into ware groups. The medieval sherds from the site were examined under x20 magnification and a fabric description recorded. The pottery was quantified by sherd count and sherd weight, the sherds being divided into rim or bodybase sherds.

A total of 142 sherds, weighing 3451g, were recovered from the site. The overwhelming majority of the sherds dated to the later 18th and 19th centuries and comprised an unexceptional mix of factory-produced wares and some coarsewares.

A number of features produced pottery of an earlier date. The excavations of four graves (HB 11, 76, 104, and 122) recovered sherds dating to the late 17th–18th century. These included coarse and blackware, yellow ware, feathered slipware, and manganese mottled ware. A single blackware mug rim was recovered from the grave containing HB 122. One pit (F216) produced sherds of yellow ware and Midlands purple coarseware. This probably represented the earliest post-medieval material and dated to the later 16th or 17th centuries. The early post-medieval pottery contained little diagnostic material.

Four contexts contained only single sherds of medieval pottery. The sherds recovered from the graves of HB 85 and 144 (contexts 1254 and 1422 respectively) are most likely residual. Two further sherds of medieval pottery were recovered from ditch F214 (context 1397) and posthole F216 (context 1399). Medieval pottery has been rarely found in Wolverhampton and for this reason the four medieval sherds are described fully here.

Context 1254
Sandy iron-rich hand-formed, ?wheel-finished, cooking pot sherd with heavy external soot. The fabric is similar to fabric F02 from Stafford Castle (Ratkai in preparation). Abundant, ill-sorted, sub-angular and sub-rounded quartz, 0.25–0.75mm.
Orange-brown external surface, brown internal surface, grey core.
Date: 13th–14th century.

Context 1397
Sandy iron-poor hand-formed, glazed body sherd.
Abundant sub-angular quartz *c* 0.5–0.75mm.
Sparse rounded red-brown, ferruginous inclusions 0.25–2mm.
Buff inner surface, pale orange external surface, buff margins.

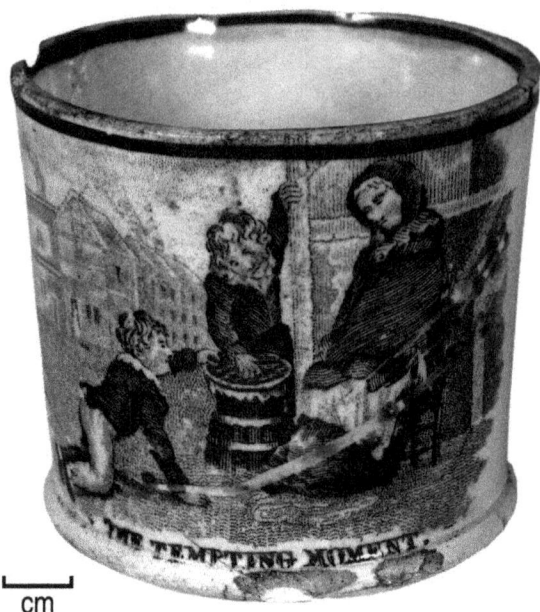

Plate 14 Earthenware pot recovered with HB 25

Pale olive glaze spots present on the external surface.
Date: mid-13th–14th century.

Context 1399
Iron-rich, wheel-thrown, glazed sherd.
Sparse sub-angular ill-sorted quartz up to 0.5mm.
Sparse rounded red-brown, ferruginous inclusions up to 0.5mm.
Sparse sub-angular off-white inclusions (no reaction to hydrochloric acid).
Sparse irregular voids *c* 0.25mm.
Orange fabric, some pale and red streaks visible within it.
Internal and external thin olive glaze.
Date: The fabric resembles a better prepared version of some of the early post-medieval coarseware fabrics. The glaze and form suggest a medieval date, the fabric a later medieval date of the 14th or, possibly, 15th century.

Context 1422
Sandy iron-rich, hand-formed, cooking pot rim sherd.
Moderate rounded and sub-rounded quartz *c* 0.25–0.5mm.
Rare (1 piece) of coarse-grained sandstone *c* 0.75mm.
The rim sherd was completely reduced, mid-grey in section with paler surfaces. The rim was everted with an expanded rounded terminal.
Date: On typological grounds, possibly 12th century but no later than the 13th century.

The fabrics were not matched exactly to other South Staffordshire pottery but they fall within the same tradition as pottery found at Dudley (personal inspection by author) and there is no reason to suppose that they were anything other than of local manufacture.

Small earthenware pot
A small printed earthenware pot with a painted band around the rim (Plate 14) was found associated with HB 25, an adult burial in an earth-cut grave. It is illustrated with a scene showing children stealing chestnuts from a brazier.

A similar image was used on a plate illustrated in *Gifts for Good Children, Part I;...1790–1890* (Riley 1991, 52–3). David Barker from the Stoke-on-Trent Archaeology Service explains that this is a fairly common type of pot produced by many potteries in Staffordshire and the Northeast from the 1820s onwards.

Items with printed patterns such as this were popular, and in some cases may have been associated with children, although not exclusively so. The burial with which the cup was associated was not that of a child.

DENTURES *by Annette Hancocks*

A single fragmentary set of vulcanite dentures was recovered from the backfill of Vault 6 (Plate 11). The roof of the vault was virtually intact, although some disturbance at the eastern end had occurred during the 1973 clearance. The dentures are well preserved but fragmentary and were recovered from a deposit associated with disarticulated bones. They compare favourably to a complete set of the late 19th century recently recovered from St Martin's Churchyard, Birmingham (Hancocks in Brickley *et al* 2006, 140), and from Christ Church, Spitalfields (Molleson 1993, 53-60).

The majority of 19th-century dentures were constructed with a mixture of natural 'Waterloo' and ceramic teeth sprung with gold spiral springs. The incomplete set of dentures recovered comprises a complete upper set of 'tubeless' tube teeth. Platinum pins were used to hold the teeth in place. Gold coil springs were a long-standing holding-in device and were attached to each denture by a rotary pin. The upper denture set recovered has the rotary pin and plate still attached to the denture with a 1cm fragment of the coil spring surviving at each fixing point. Additionally, there is some damage to the dentures on the upper left palate, which has left the platinum pins exposed. Also of note on this upper denture is a 'D'-shaped indentation, which would create suction, allowing the denture to be held in place to the roof of the mouth. Only half of the lower left denture plate survives. A single 1cm fragment of coil spring survives, which is fixed into the denture by a rotary pin.

The British Dental Association Museum houses an excellent reference collection and holds documentation of the processes of manufacture, fitting and maintenance (Tomes 1851).

Table 7 Quantities of coffin furniture

	Quantity (number)	Quantity (weight in grams)
Coffin handles (grips)	208	57372
Coffin plate	2688	26401
Coffin nails	471	1044

Manufacturing process using the high pressure vulcanizing oven

A beeswax cast would be taken of the profile of the individual mouth. This would form the basis of a mould for casting the dentures. Vulcanite would be the casting solution. Porcelain teeth of the size and shape best suited to the patient's need were mounted in pink wax as trial dentures that could be checked in the mouth for appearance and function.

The wax trial dentures were embedded in plaster in a metal flask (ie box) and the wax washed away with boiling water. The tinted rubber/ sulphur mix, brown for the base, pink for the gum, was packed between and around the porcelain teeth. The flask, when filled, was clamped and subjected to 100lb steam pressure, at about 160 °C, for approximately two hours.

After the flask had cooled, the denture was separated from the plaster, trimmed with files and scrapers and polished.

COFFIN FURNITURE by Emma Hancox

A total of 16 boxes of coffin furniture were recovered from the excavations. The furniture consisted mostly of grips (handles), grip plates, *depositum* plates and nails from the coffins (Table 7). The majority of the assemblage came from the earth-cut graves, with the remainder coming from the vaults. The fragmentary remains of at least 18 coffins were identified.

The material was dated, stylistically, from the mid-18th to the late 19th century, mostly from *c* 1830–1880. This corresponds well with the probable time period over which the cemetery was used. There were problems with residuality and contamination. The vaults had been mostly cleared in 1973 and back filled with modern debris. This resulted in disarticulated bone and coffin furniture being scattered across the floors of the vaults. The furniture could not always be related to a body, or even in some cases to the vault, as it could have been thrown in during the clearance. The material from the grave cuts also suffers from residuality. In some cases the material from the fills may not be associated with the burial in the cut, but may be from earlier burials in the same area.

The preservation of the majority of the assemblage is poor. The grips are mostly too corroded to assess the shape, or see any decoration, and most of the plates are extremely fragmented. Two legible *depositum* plates survived in association with bodies and some of the grip plates from the vaults still had identifiable patterns.

Prior to 1700, coffins were trapezoidal in shape with gable lids, sometimes with handles, of the type found on domestic furniture (Litten 1991, 99). Around the turn of the 18th century, the funerary trade underwent a dramatic change, with funerals and all their accoutrements becoming much more elaborate. From this time the vast majority of coffins became single break (a few were rectangular) and flat lidded with up to three shells of wood and lead. They tended to be adorned with a variety of grips, grip plates, *depositum* plates, hatchment plates, and eschuteons. All the coffins at St Peter's, where identified, were single break, flat lidded and highly decorated. They were definitely all post-1750 in style, and the majority appeared to be from 1830–1880. Of the patterns on the grip plates, the 'winged cherub' and a floral motif were the only ones identified. The cherub motif dates from *c* 1743–1847 (Patrick 2001, 7) and is found on most post-medieval sites and at all levels of society (Boore 1998, 73).

Only one triple-shell lead coffin was recorded. This was in Vault 7, which was the only vault which appeared to be uncontaminated by the grave clearance. Five other coffins were found in this vault, recorded as wood and metal coffins. Only five grips and 79g of plate were kept from this vault. They were all very corroded and fragmented.

WOOD REMAINS FROM COFFINS by Rowena Gale

This report includes the assessment of six samples of coffin wood recovered during the excavation. The samples examined related to Vaults 1, 3, 5 and 7, and the earth-cut grave containing HB 80.

Each sample consisted of several pieces of wood, all of which were poorly preserved and degraded; mostly, these were still damp, although some were dry. The samples were prepared for examination using standard methods for waterlogged and desiccated wood (Gale and Cutler 2000). Thin sections were removed from the damp timber from the transverse, tangential and radial surfaces and mounted on microscope slides. These were examined at magnifications up to x400 using transmitted light on a Nikon Labophot-2 compound microscope. For desiccated wood, newly exposed (fractured) surfaces in similar orientations were supported in sand and examined using incident light illumination on the same microscope. The anatomical structure was matched to reference material

Table 8 Identification of coffin woods

Vault	Description of strat unit	Human burial	Identification and comments
001	coffin	5	1 x elm (*Ulmus* sp.), heartwood
			3 x pine (*Pinus* sp.), Scots pine group (*sylvestris* group)
003	coffin	-	Several pieces from wide panel/ plank, elm (*Ulmus* sp.), heartwood
003	coffin	7	Several pieces, oak (*Quercus* sp.), heartwood
005	coffin	14	2 x oak (*Quercus* sp.), heartwood
			3 x spruce (*Picea*) or larch (*Larix*)
007	coffin	42	Several pieces of oak (*Quercus* sp.), heartwood
	coffin	90	Thin slivers of elm (*Ulmus* sp.), heartwood

(Table 8). Where possible, the maturity of the wood was assessed (ie heartwood/ sapwood).

Evidence from the wood analysis indicates the use of at least four types of timber associated with the construction of the coffins. The taxa identified are shown on Table 8 and listed below.

Elm (*Ulmus* sp.)
Oak (*Quercus* sp.)
Pine (*Pinus* sp.), Scots pine group (*sylvestris* group)
Spruce (*Picea*) or larch (*Larix*); these taxa are anatomically similar.

Oak and elm timbers are very durable when underground, pine slightly less so; all three taxa have probably been more frequently used than any other species for coffin making over the last few centuries (Edlin 1949). Coffins HB 5 (Vault 1) and HB 14 (Vault 5) included two wood types (elm and pine, and oak and spruce/ larch, respectively) but it is not known how these woods were distributed in the make-up of the coffins or, indeed, whether some of the wood derived from coffin supports or other components, rather than the actual coffins.

With regard to the spruce/ larch identification it is not usually possible to distinguish between these genera using anatomical features. Larch is extremely durable in damp or wet conditions whereas spruce is very perishable (Lincoln 1986) and it might, therefore, be assumed that larch was more likely to have been used. Interestingly, however, Lincoln (*ibid*) records the commercial use of spruce, not larch, for coffins.

It is probable that coffin makers obtained the bulk of their timber from local sources. Oak and elm are both indigenous and suitably wide boards were probably easily obtained. Softwoods such as pine (probably Scots pine in this instance, known commercially as redwood) and spruce/ larch could either have been imported or obtained from British plantations. Although native stocks of Scots

pine have been more or less confined to Scotland since prehistoric times, it was introduced into cultivation in England in recent centuries as a garden specimen and on a commercial basis for timber. Pine timber was imported to Britain from the Baltic from at least the 12th century (Rackham 1986). Neither spruce nor larch are native but were introduced into cultivation in the late 14th and 17th centuries respectively (Mitchell 1974), and have formed an important aspect of the timber trade.

Since the families or individuals owning the vaults and grave are unknown it has not been possible to correlate the use of specific timbers with status, age or gender.

The wood samples probably derive from wide planks and, as such, represent trees of unknown and possibly considerable age. The wood was too degraded or fragmented to assess whether it was likely to have originated from inner or outer areas of the trunk.

Spruce (*Picea*), larch (*Larix*) and pine (*Pinus sp.*) are comparatively short-lived, especially when grown for timber, but none the less, these samples could be up to a century or so in age. Oak (*Quercus sp.*) and elm (*Ulmus sp.*) both have natural life spans of some centuries, although oak will usually out-live elm.

In view of the absence of short-lived material, the comparative modernity of the site and the lack of documentation for the individuals interred, radiocarbon dating was not undertaken.

The current wood analysis has identified the use of a range of timbers, both native and non-native, for coffin making in early to mid-19th-century Wolverhampton. While the lack of documentary evidence prevents comparison of use between individual burials, the details obtained are of significance on a broader scale in establishing a database of 19th-century funerary practices in the region.

CHAPTER 5

Skeletal Analysis

Iraia Arabaolaza, Paola Ponce, Anthea Boylston

Anthropological analysis of the skeletal assemblage recovered from the excavations was undertaken. Various techniques and methodologies were used to assess the assemblage for physical anthropology, including minimum number of individuals, bone preservation, age and sex, stature, cranial index, and non-metric traits. Dental health and disease was investigated, as was skeletal pathology. The crude prevalence rates for a number of diseases and conditions from this assemblage were then compared to a similar data set from excavations at St Martin's in Birmingham (Brickley *et al* 2006).

PHYSICAL ANTHROPOLOGY

Table 9 Minimum number of individuals (articulated adults)

Side	Right	Left	Unsided
Medial clavicle	41	35	0
Lateral clavicle	36	36	0
Proximal humerus	45	48	0
Distal humerus	55	51	0
Proximal ulna	57	51	0
Distal ulna	43	39	0
Proximal radius	49	40	0
Distal radius	48	43	0
Proximal femur	46	45	0
Distal femur	41	42	0
Proximal tibia	31	35	0
Distal tibia	26	23	0
Proximal fibula	13	12	0
Distal fibula	15	18	0
Patella	28	37	0
Frontal	51	52	0
Occipital	0	0	55
Temporal	54	54	0
Calcaneus	26	27	0
Talus	27	28	0
Foot	35	33	0
Os-coxae	48	48	0
Sacrum	0	0	41
Manubrium	0	0	33
Sternum	0	0	34
Ribs	64	65	0
Scapula	52	48	0
Hands	61	59	0

Minimum number of individuals

Archaeologically, 152 burials were recorded, although subsequent anthropological analysis revealed 150

articulated skeletons. Some burials, which were considered to contain a single individual, included sufficient additional skeletal material to be judged as another separate individual. In most of these cases the same number was given to the additional skeletal elements, but with an additional suffix (eg HB 12a and 12b). Anatomical elements were counted in order to calculate a minimum number of individuals (MNI) for the articulated burials (Tables 9 and 10).

Table 10 Minimum number of individuals (articulated subadults)

Side	Right	Left	Unsided
Medial clavicle	27	26	0
Lateral clavicle	23	20	0
Proximal humerus	29	25	0
Distal humerus	25	25	0
Proximal ulna	28	25	0
Distal ulna	19	18	0
Proximal radius	22	24	0
Distal radius	20	20	0
Proximal fémur	34	29	0
Distal fémur	26	22	0
Proximal tibia	19	19	0
Distal tibia	19	17	0
Proximal fibula	14	14	0
Distal fibula	12	13	0
Patella	5	5	0
Frontal	29	29	0
Occipital	0	0	33
Temporal	33	33	0
Calcaneus	10	12	0
Talus	11	10	0
Foot	17	15	0
Os-coxae	33	29	0
Sacrum	0	0	28
Manubrium	0	0	16
Sternum	0	0	21
Ribs	41	41	0
Scapula	31	30	0
Hands	22	23	0

Some of the skeletal material identified in discrete burials at the time of excavation (HB 8, 9 and 10, and HB 33) was considered to be disarticulated due to the number of intrusive animal and human bones present in the grave fill. Further disarticulated material was recovered from unstratified contexts across the site. All of the

Table 11   Minimum number of individuals (disarticulated material)

Side	Right	Left	Unsided	Fragments
Clavicle	7	10	0	2
Distal humerus	22	14	0	35
Proximal ulna	5	8	0	37
Distal radius	9	4	0	26
Proximal femur	16	17	0	5
Distal femur	10	9	0	53
Proximal tibia	4	4	0	37
Distal tibia	14	7	0	0
Distal fibula	4	3	0	18
Maxilla	0	0	0	2
Mandible	0	0	0	8
Frontal	0	0	0	3
Occipital	0	0	0	18
Temporal	11	15	0	0
Tarsals	0	0	25	9
Metatarsals	0	0	67	7
Phalanges	0	0	49	0
Os-coxae	3	1	70	0
Ilium	11	8	0	0
Ischium	11	6	0	0
Pubis	0	10	0	0
Manubrium	0	0	6	0
Sternum	0	0	7	0
Scapula	7	5	27	0
Carpals	13	9	0	1
Metacarpals	42	24	0	9
Phalanges	0	0	67	12

disarticulated material was combined, and certain anatomical points were counted, to establish the MNI. In the case of adult skeletal elements, the most frequently occurring were the right distal humerus (22) and the left proximal femur (17). For juvenile disarticulated remains, the most common elements were also the right humerus (9) and the left femur (10) (Tables 11 and 12). The disarticulated remains contained a minimum of 22 adults and ten juveniles.

Table 13   Preservation categories

Preservation	Total	Percentage
Excellent	18	12.16%
Good	53	35.81%
Fair	59	39.86%
Poor	18	12.16%

Table 14   Completeness categories

Completeness	Total	Percentage
< 25 %	50	33.78 %
25-50 %	23	15.54 %
50-75 %	39	26.35 %
75 + %	36	24.32 %

Table 12   Minimum number of individuals (disarticulated material from subadults)

Side	Right	Left	Unsided	Fragments	Age Categories
Clavicle	0	0	4	0	2 inf, 2 YC
Humerus	9	3	0	7	4 inf, 4 YC, 1 OC
Ulna	1	2	0	0	1 inf, 2 C
Radius	0	0	4	0	2 inf, 2 C
Femur	2	10	1	1	3 inf, 6 YC, 1 OC
Tibia	7	7	1	0	3 inf, 5 YC, 1 OC
Fibula	0	0	7	0	2 inf, 4 C, 1 ADO
Maxilla	0	0	2	0	2 YC
Mandible	0	0	6	0	1 inf, 5 YC
Cranium	0	0	0	95	
Metatarsals	0	0	6	2	6 OC
Phalanges	0	0	2	0	
Ilium	3	3	4	0	1 inf, 2 YC, 1 OC
Pubis	0	0	1	0	1 YC
Sacrum	0	0	2	0	
Vertebra	0	0	25	0	
Scapula	4	0	0	0	3 inf, 1 YC

Preservation

The quality and quantity of information that a burial collection can provide depends on the preservation of the skeletal remains. Preservation is related to both the completeness of the skeleton (completeness) and quality of the skeletal material found (degree of preservation). Despite the high level of later disturbance on this site, the degree of preservation of the human bones was good. Half of the human burials fell into 'excellent' or 'good' degree of preservation (Table 13), that is to say the bone surface was in a good state, without any erosion of the cortical bone. Hair was still remaining on some of the crania and/ or mandibles of ten individuals (HB 25, 26, 37, 41, 47, 51, 61, 67, 101, and 102). The number of fairly complete skeletons was also high; half of them were placed in the 50–75% complete or more than 75% complete category (Table 14). The presence of skeletons allocated to the least complete category is some indication of the degree of disturbance during the later clearance and construction works.

Age and sex estimation

The assessment of age at death separated the individuals into adult and juvenile categories. The age of 18 was taken as a cut-off point, because by this age eruption of the third molars and fusion of the long bones epiphyses is usually complete. Of the 150 articulated skeletons analysed, 58 were juveniles and 92 were adults.

After this general classification, standard age estimation techniques were applied to the material in order to get a more precise age range. This system subdivided juveniles into six groups: fetus (under 40 weeks), neonate (birth–1 month), infant (1 month–12 months), early childhood (1–6 years), late childhood (7–12 years), and adolescent (13–17 years). In addition, adults were subdivided in four groups: young adult (18–25 years), young middle adult (26–35), old middle adult (36–45, and mature adult (46+). In some cases, where the preservation or completeness of the individuals did not allow ageing techniques to be applied, only the adult or juvenile category was given to the skeleton.

Age estimation

The accuracy of age-at-death estimates depends on the preservation and completeness of the skeleton, as this affects the number of diagnostic skeletal elements that can be used in the estimation of age. However, it is

important to bear in mind that the age obtained is biological and not chronological, so ten-year age groups are the most precise age-at-death estimate that can be obtained for adults (Waldron 1994).

The techniques employed for ageing the adult skeleton were: changes in the morphology of the pubic symphysis (Todd 1921a, 1921b; Brooks and Suchey 1990); changes in the morphology of the auricular surface (Lovejoy *et al* 1985; Meindl and Lovejoy 1989); closure of the vault and the lateral-anterior cranial sutures (Meindl and Lovejoy 1985); and morphological changes in the sternal end of the fourth rib (Iscan *et al* 1984; 1985). In some instances, the ossification of the thyroid cartilage (Krogman and Iscan 1986, 128) was used to assess the age category, which was particularly useful for estimating the age of the oldest individuals.

The age estimation techniques for juveniles were: tooth eruption (Ubelaker 1989, 63–5) and developmental stages (Moorrees *et al* 1963a; 1963b), epiphyseal fusion (Scheuer and Black 2004), and long bone length (Scheuer and Black 2000; Sundick 1978; Ubelaker 1989, 65–71). The most reliable methods were tooth developmental stages and tooth eruption. For long bone length, the measurements taken from Scheuer and Black (2000) were the most accurate for this study as they were based mainly on British populations. Additionally, the age estimates obtained using Scheuer and Black's long bone length measurements were similar to the age ranges obtained from the two dental methods (Table 15).

Sex estimation

As for age estimation, assessment of sex of a skeleton is dependent on its level of preservation and completeness. In the case of juveniles, sex assessment is very complicated as features that differentiate between males and females start to develop during adolescence. Most of the juveniles were categorised as skeletons of indeterminate sex, with the exception of four adolescent individuals who were sexed using the morphological characteristics used to estimate the sex of the adults (Table 16).

The adult sex estimation methods used were based principally on the morphological differences of the skull and pelvic region, which are sexually dimorphic. The pelvis is the most accurate zone for sex estimation

Table 15 The number of individuals in each age category

Sub-adult <18	Young Adult 18-25	Young Middle Adult 26-35	Old Middle Adult 36-45	Mature Adult 46+	Adult 18+	Total
58	5	13	26	23	25	150
38.6%	3.3%	8.6%	17.3%	15.3%	16.6%	100%

Table 16   Age and sex categories of the sample

Age Category	Male	? Male	Female	? Female	Indeterminate
Fetus Neonatal Infant Early Childhood Late Childhood Adolescent		 1		 3	2 1 25 18 4 4
Young Adult	1	1	3	0	0
Young Middle Adult	3	2	7	1	0
Old Middle Adult	14	2	9	0	1
Mature Adult	9	0	12	2	0
Adult	3	3	1	3	15

Table 17   The number of individuals in each sex category

Male	Male?	Female	Female?	Indeterminate	Total
30	9	32	9	70	150

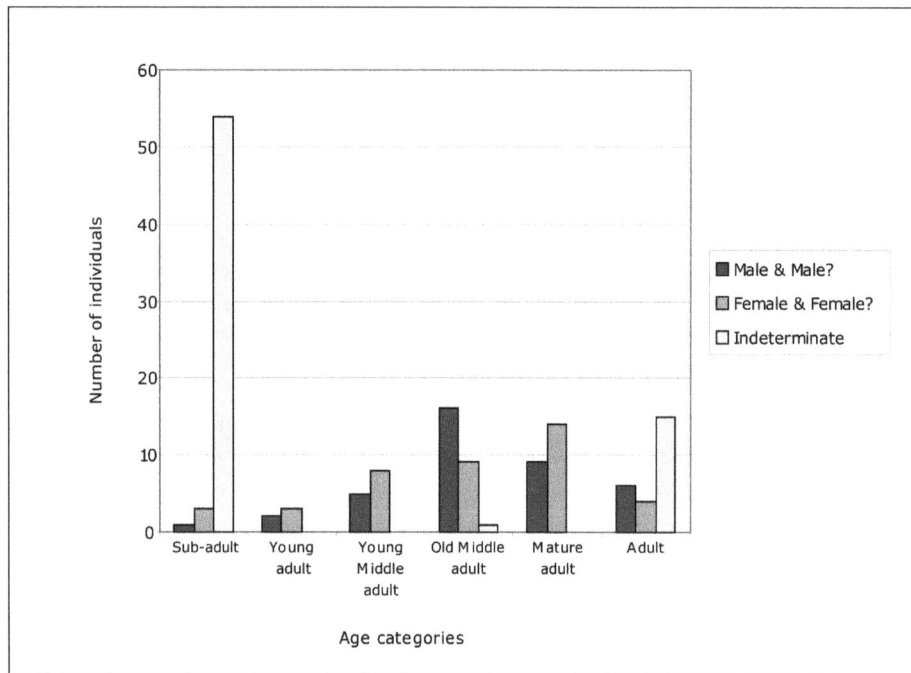

Figure 11 Demographic profile of burials

(Ubelaker 1989 53). The morphological traits of the pelvis observed for this population were: the ventral arc, subpubic concavity, subpubic angle, ischio-pubic ramus ridge, greater sciatic notch, preauricular sulcus, obturator foramen, acetabulum, pelvic brim, sacral segments, and sacral morphology (Bass 1987). In addition, the skull features examined were: the nuchal crest, mastoid process, posterior zygomatic arch, supraorbital margin, supraorbital ridge, glabella, parietal bossing, frontal bossing, mental eminence, gonial angle, gonial flaring, mandibular ramus, and palate shape. All of these features were scored following criteria outlined in Buikstra and Ubelaker (1994). Alongside these features, metrical assessment of sex using the maximum clavicle length, glenoid cavity width, humeral head diameter, radial head diameter, femoral head diameter and femoral bicondylar width were used (Stewart 1979).

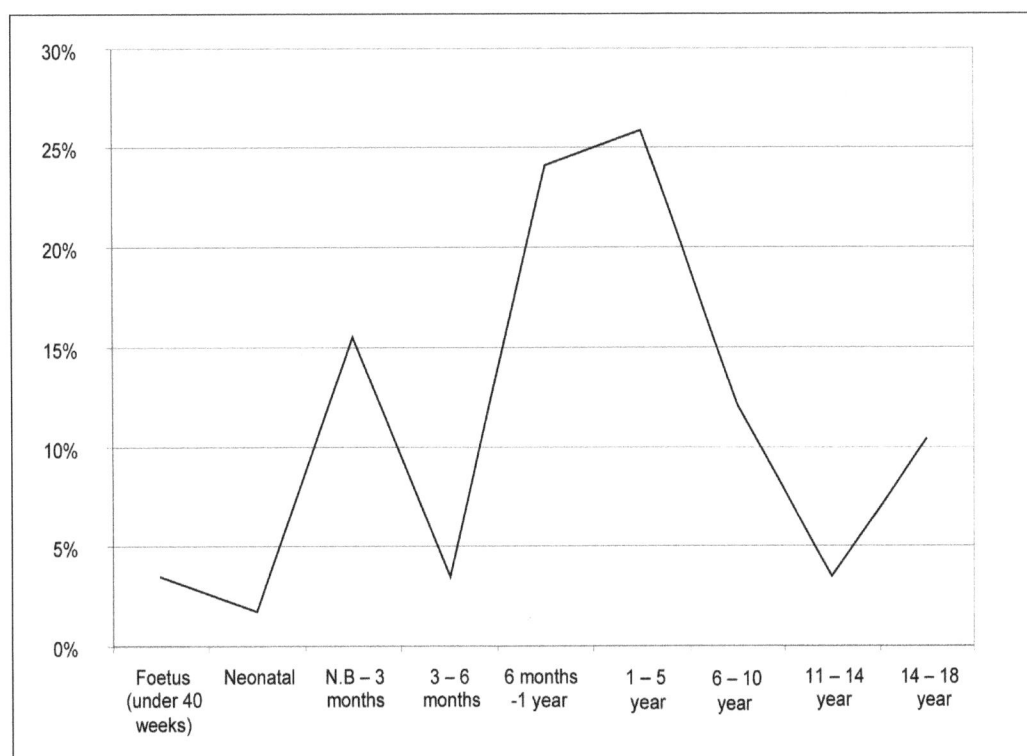

Figure 12 Percentage of sub-adult deaths by age group

As the results in Table 17 demonstrate, the sex ratio of this population was normal, with almost equal numbers of males and females. In addition, the high frequency of individuals of indeterminate sex is due to the elevated number of juveniles and to some poorly preserved skeletons within the sample studied.

The demographic profile of this population has a 'U' shaped distribution (Fig 11). Nearly 40% of the entire population were juveniles, a similar demographic profile to that obtained for St Bride's Lower Churchyard, London (Bowman *et al* 1993). Analysing the juveniles according to their age-at-death category indicates that the peak in mortality occurred between six months and five years (Fig 12). This could be related to the hazards associated with weaning. In the Victorian period it was very fashionable to feed the growing infant with 'pap' or 'panada' (a mixture of water and flour), which led to defective nutrition resulting in a poor immune system. As a result, children of weaning age were at a higher risk of contracting diseases, and gastro-intestinal infections in particular (Lewis 2002, 10–11; Roberts and Cox 2003, 307). Other archaeological sites from this period with high infant mortality associated with weaning include Christ Church Spitalfields, London (Molleson *et al* 1993, 183).

Stature
Estimation of stature was made for those adult individuals who had intact long bones (humerus, radius, ulna, femur, tibia, and fibula) using the formulae developed by Trotter (1970). The most reliable result for this technique is when the femur and tibia measurements are combined; however, in this report all the limb bones were used. When both sides were present, the longer measurement was used to estimate stature (Table 18).

As the results in Table 19 demonstrate, the estimated statures, for both males and females from the site, fall within the range of stature estimates from other contemporary sites, including Christ Church Spitalfields, London (Molleson *et al* 1993), or Redcross Way, London (Brickley and Miles 1999). Although the Christ Church Spitalfields burials were derived from a wealthier population, the mean stature and range obtained for St Peter's was slightly higher, especially when comparing the results from the females. However, this difference could be due to the longer period of use of the Spitalfields crypt or the wider range of the results obtained from St Peter's where the standard deviation was 5.37 for males and 5.20 for females.

Table 18   Stature (cm)

Sex	Mean	Range	Standard deviation (SD)	No of individuals
Male	171.0	161.7 – 181.3	5.37	30
Female	160.6	150.4 – 173	5.20	25

Table 19   Intersite stature comparison

Site	Period	Male			Female		
	Century	Mean (cm)	Range (cm)	n	Mean (cm)	Range (cm)	n
St Peter's Wolverhampton (this study)	mid-19th	171.0	161.7-181.3	30	160.6	150.4-173	25
Redcross Way	mid-19th	168.5	153-180	16	158.2	142-172	19
St Bride's Lower Churchyard	Post-medieval	171.1	150-191	-	156.8	143-171	-
Christ Church,* Spitalfields	18th- mid 19th	167.9 - 170.3	-	-	154 - 158.5	-	-

*Results obtained from Brickley *et al* 1999

Table 20 Cranial measurements

Measurement	Male					Female				
	m	sd	min	max	n	m	sd	min	max	n
Cranial length	189.9	6.58	178	135	12	183	9.15	170	199	16
Cranial breadth	143.4	4.62	135	153	14	134.5	6.50	120	148	13
Bizygomatic diameter	129.3	6.02	119	136	7	119.4	4.72	115	127	5
Basion-bregma height	137.5	7.90	123	155	15	136.6	4.84	131	145	10
Cranial base length	100.7	17.08	49	117	12	107.2	18.05	91	145	11
Biauricular breadth	126.6	8.52	112	141	14	114.9	7.19	101	125	12
Minimum frontal breadth	102.5	8.91	91	118	13	99.8	7.28	92	114	19
Upper facial breadth	106.6	4.06	98	111	11	102.3	3.77	96	110	17
Upper facial height	70.6	6.60	58	82	10	77.2	17.89	66	113	6
Nasal height	52.7	2.87	47	57	9	52.6	4.39	48	59	5
Nasal breadth	24.3	1.82	21	28	12	22.7	2.16	20	26	6
Orbital height	35.4	2.67	31	39	8	34.0	1.87	32	36	5
Orbital breadth	42.4	3.09	37	47	12	71.7	4.62	38	53	10
Maxillo-alveolar length	54.7	3.73	49	63	12	49.7	4.68	45	56	6
Maxillo-alveolar breadth	57.2	4.76	49	63	12	54.3	3.15	52	61	7
Frontal chord	114.6	8.05	98	130	14	112.9	4.59	103	120	19
Parietal chord	118.1	7.13	108	135	19	114.8	8.22	95	128	17
Occipital chord	98.7	10.20	77	124	18	87.4	16.51	57	118	12
Bicondylar breadth	123.9	7.79	114	140	9	109.8	3.56	106	115	5
Bigonial breadth	103.5	6.46	93	115	12	93.6	9.49	84	122	13
Minimum ramus breadth	33.2	3.00	27	38	24	28.2	3.01	24	35	18
Symphyseal height	31.8	3.91	24	41	24	26.6	3.68	21	32	20

Population variability

Standard anthropological measurements were taken of the cranium and post-cranial skeleton in order to analyse variability both within the population and between different contemporary skeletal assemblages (Bass 1987, 61). The variation in the skull and/ or post-cranial bones is related to environmental and genetic factors (Brothwell 1981), nutrition and diet (Mays 1998). All the measurements (Tables 20 and 21) were taken from intact and non-pathological bones to reduce the risk of errors.

Cranial index

Cranial indices provide information relating to the evolution of human head shape. These have shown that medieval populations had a broader head compared with populations from the 17th–19th centuries (Goose 1981). These dissimilarities could be related to differences in diet (Luther 1993). The cranial indices for the St Peter's population illustrate that there was a difference in cranial shape between males, mostly mesocranial (average head), and females, which fell into the dolichocranial category (long head). However, the disparity between the sexes was less when the means were studied (Table 22). The height and length index for both sexes, males 73.7 and females 74.6, fell within average measurements (Bass 1987). This was not the case for the breadth and height index, where males fell into the average category (96.5), but females were found to have a higher skull (101.7).

Table 21 Postcranial measurements

Measurement	Male					Female				
	mean	min	max	sd	n	mean	min	max	sd	n
Right clavicle length	154.4	133	166	7.7	13	135.3	114	151	8.6	16
Left clavicle length	150.0	130	164	9.8	11	137.1	131	145	4.6	9
Right glenoid cavity width	28.4	25	31	2.0	15	24.4	22	27	1.8	17
Left glenoid cavity width	28	24	31	2.2	12	23.9	22	28	1.6	12
Right humeral length	328.7	304	356	15.1	12	306	281	326	13.8	14
Left humeral length	328.6	306	349	12.2	11	298	284	320	13.4	12
Right Hum head diameter	46.5	42	51	3.0	14	41.3	39	47	2.0	14
Left Hum head diameter	47.6	42	53	3.1	13	40.7	38	46	2.0	14
Right Hum bicondylar width	63.6	59	72	3.3	21	56.7	51	66	3.9	18
Left Hum bicondylar width	63.4	59	68	2.6	17	55.7	51	67	4.0	19
Right max diam at midshaft	21.8	17	26	2.4	25	19.9	15	23	1.9	21
Left max diam at midshaft	21.2	17	27	2.4	24	19	15	21	1.6	26
Right radial length	240.1	222	258	11.4	15	219.2	203	236	10.4	11
Left radial length	235.4	193	256	16.1	13	223.5	196	250	16.8	10
Right max head diameter	24	21	27	1.6	19	21.1	19	25	1.5	17
Left max head diameter	23.6	20	27	1.6	14	21.1	19	24	1.4	14
Right ulnar length	259.8	245	287	11.9	15	238	222	260	13.4	11
Left ulnar length	256.6	234	275	14.2	10	238.6	218	260	11.5	13
Right femoral length	467.1	432	499	20.7	11	428.1	390	457	17.6	11
Left femoral length	458.6	425	488	21.3	16	424.2	392	445	16.5	13
Right femur bicondylar length	470.6	436	503	20.8	10	427.0	394	458	17.2	11
Left femur bicondylar length	458.3	424	493	21.9	16	422.3	390	440	16.1	13
Right femoral head diameter	48.5	42	54	2.8	24	42.8	38	48	2.3	17
Left femoral head diameter	48.7	43	54	2.8	19	42.7	39	47	2.3	18
Right A-P diameter	29.8	25	36	3.3	23	27.6	19	35	3.1	19
Left A-P diameter	30.0	26	35	2.2	21	27	23	30	1.8	19
Right M-L diameter	33.7	29	39	2.6	23	30.4	24	34	2.2	19
Left M-L diameter	33.6	30	37	1.9	21	30.3	28	38	2.4	19
Right midshaft A-P diameter	29.3	27	32	1.5	24	26.7	19	30	2.4	21
Left midshaft A-P diameter	29.7	27	38	2.4	22	27	24	30	1.7	21
Right midshaft M-L diameter	28.0	24	33	2.2	24	25.7	22	30	1.7	21
Left midshaft M-L diameter	28.2	24	32	2.0	22	25.8	23	31	2.0	21
Right bicondylar width	83.5	75	91	4.3	15	73.3	70	79	3.1	10
Left bicondylar width	83.5	75	93	4.8	14	73.3	70	79	3.2	12
Right tibial length	378.3	330	412	26.2	10	342.8	317	355	15.3	5
Left tibial length	375.6	326	398	26.6	8	346.1	318	359	14.2	7
Right prox.epiphyseal	75.9	67	87	6.2	11	71.8	66	95	8.4	10

breadth										
Left prox epiphyseal breadth	75.3	66	82	6.0	10	69.2	66	74	2.6	8
Right A-P diameter	35.4	31	40	2.6	14	30.6	29	34	1.9	9
Left A-P diameter	35.7	33	41	2.5	17	30.1	23	34	3.0	14
Right M-L diameter	26.2	23	30	1.6	14	22.7	21	24	1.2	9
Left M-L diameter	26.0	23	30	2.2	17	23.5	20	32	2.9	14
Right fibular length	366.3	332	385	29.7	3	314				1
Left fibular length	386.3	382	389	3.5	3	338				1

Table 22 Indices

Index	Male					Female				
	m	sd	min	max	n	m	sd	min	max	n
Cranial	75.2	2.29	72.1	78.3	11	73.9	3.42	66.3	78.7	13
Cranial length / height	73.7	2.80	70.1	78.4	12	74.6	4.45	65.8	82.9	11
Cranial Breadth / height	96.5	4.83	84.3	102.9	13	101.7	7.08	90.5	117.5	10
Mean height										
Fronto-parietal	71.7	4.95	65.7	79.2	10	72.8	5.50	66.7	85.8	12
Nasal	46.7	6.16	38.9	59.6	9	42.2	6.13	33.9	50.0	5
Total facial										
Upper facial	55.0	4.03	47.4	60.3	7	60.4	1.89	58.3	62.5	4
Orbital	83.5	7.12	73.9	95.1	8	86.4	5.35	82.0	92.3	5
Maxillo-alveolar	106.6	86.7	121.2	12.31	11	110	8.99	92.9	117.8	6

One of the male skulls (HB 119, a young adult) had morphological traits consistent with a mixed racial ancestry. His cranium was dolichocranial and, even though his height/ length index was close to the male mean pattern, his breadth/ height index was high in relation to the rest of the population. The skull had more features in common with the female population than the male. However, this diversity could be characteristic of the racial ancestry of this individual.

Post-cranial measurements
The post-cranial measurements taken (Table 21) were used to calculate stature and determine the sex of the individual. Although the platymeric and platycnemic indices were estimated, these did not reveal any significant trends.

Non–metric traits
As suggested by their name, these traits are not measurable but reveal information about population variability and activity through variations in the morphology of bone (Brothwell 1981). Some non-metric traits relate to genetic factors, whereas other traits are associated with the environment, occupation and lifestyle of the individual (Brickley and Miles 1999). Non-metric traits were scored as either present or absent using the diagrams provided by Berry and Berry (1967) for the cranium and Finnegan (1978) for the post-cranial bones. Evidence for a metopic suture was recorded on 11% of crania and nearly half the crania analysed exhibited lambdoidal wormian bones. Looking at the foramina,

37% showed supra-orbital foramina and 54% parietal foramina. Ossicles at the parietal notch were recorded on 7% of the skulls. The most common non-metric trait in the post-cranial skeleton was the double anterior calcaneal facet, with almost 40% of the calcanei involved. Double inferior talar facets were the next most common (18%). Vastus notches were observed in 7.6% of total patellae. Septal aperture, on the other hand, only showed an incidence of 5.6%. Lumbar sacralisation was observed in two individuals (4.8%) and complete *spina bifida occulta* was present in one (2.4%).

Dental health and disease
During the mid-19th century, improvements in dental treatment occurred as a result of the training of dentists and the foundation of the first dental hospital in 1858 (Molleson *et al* 1993, 49), although many dentists were inexperienced and untrained. The attitudes of the general public to oral hygiene also changed, including an increased awareness of the benefits of cleaning one's teeth (rubbing them with whitening products) – although this itself sometimes damaged tooth enamel (Roberts and Cox 2003). Dental health remained poor for the working classes, due to poor diet and a lack of dental treatment. Tooth extraction was a common practice, as was the production of artificial dentures. One fragmented set of artificial vulcanite dentures (typical for this time period) was found with the disarticulated material from Vault 6 (Plate 11), indicating that at least some of the people buried at St Peter's had access to some kind of dental treatment.

Table 23   Numbers of permanent teeth available for observation (both sides combined)

	Male & ? Male		Female & ? Female		Unsexed		Tot
	max	man	max	man	max	man	
I1	13	9	11	3	2	0	38
I1	7	35	21	25	14	14	116
I2	37	42	26	31	15	14	165
C	40	45	29	36	12	11	173
PM 1	33	42	25	32	12	10	154
PM 2	31	39	21	29	9	9	138
M1	30	33	23	17	39	37	179
M2	26	32	19	15	15	10	117
M3	24	31	17	17	7	6	102
Tot	228	299	181	202	123	111	1144

Table 24   Numbers of deciduous teeth available for observation (both sides combined)

Tooth	Maxilla	Mandible	Total
I1	36	37	73
I2	34	40	74
C	40	38	78
M1	44	51	95
M2	41	47	88
Total	195	213	408

Table 25   Numbers of permanent teeth lost post mortem (both sides combined)

Tooth	Male		Female		Unsexed		Total
	max	man	max	man	max	man	
I1	13	9	11	3	2	0	38
I2	4	5	6	1	0	0	16
C	3	2	7	4	0	0	16
PM1	6	3	4	3	0	0	16
PM2	6	2	4	2	0	0	14
M1	2	3	1	2	0	0	8
M2	5	3	4	4	0	0	16
M3	4	6	3	2	0	0	15
Total	43	33	40	21	2	0	139

Table 27   Numbers of permanent teeth lost ante mortem (both sides combined)

Tooth	Male & ? Male		Female & ? Female		Unsexed	Total
	max	man	max	man	man	
I1	7	5	8	16	0	36
I2	7	3	6	13	0	29
C	6	4	4	7	0	21
PM1	10	8	7	8	0	33
PM2	11	9	13	12	0	45
M1	16	16	13	25	1	71
M2	15	17	11	23	0	66
M3	11	12	7	16	0	46
Total	83	74	69	120	1	347

Table 26   Numbers of deciduous teeth lost post mortem (both sides combined)

Tooth	Maxilla	Mandible	Total
I1	5	4	9
I2	4	1	5
C	6	2	8
M1	2	2	4
M2	3	3	6
Total	20	12	32

The preservation of the teeth in this skeletal assemblage was excellent, since teeth, due to their composition, are usually well preserved in archaeological material. A total of 1144 permanent teeth were recorded from the surviving maxillae and mandibles, as well as loose teeth (Table 23). The number of deciduous teeth recorded was also high, 408 teeth overall (Table 24). Tables 25 and 26 indicate that 139 permanent and 32 deciduous teeth were lost post mortem. By contrast, 347 permanent and 36 deciduous teeth were lost ante mortem (Tables 27 and 28). These teeth were probably lost as a result of periodontal disease, the deliberate removal of teeth or advanced age.

Analysis of calculus (tartar), dental enamel hypoplasia, abscesses, caries and periodontal disease was carried out for all the preserved teeth. Dental wear and congenital abnormalities were also examined in order to obtain a complete picture of the dentition. Individuals were sorted according to their sex and age in order to identify any

Table 28   Numbers of deciduous teeth lost ante mortem (both sides combined)

Tooth	Maxilla	Mandible	Total
I1	6	6	12
I2	6	6	12
C	3	2	5
M1	3	2	5
M2	1	1	2
Total	19	17	36

relationship between dental pathologies and sex and/ or age category. As Table 29 illustrates, females had a significantly higher prevalence of caries than males (p<0.001). In contrast, males exhibited higher rates of calculus and enamel hypoplasia.

Caries

Tooth decay, also known as dental caries, is destruction of the tooth caused by acids present in the mouth, which are produced by bacteria in the presence of sugar. These are concentrated around deposits of dental plaque, which adhere to the tooth. The frequency of dental caries increases through history, although the condition was present in early hominids (Brothwell 1981). During the 19th century, refined flours, fermentable carbohydrates and the high consumption of sugar resulted in a sharp rise in the prevalence of caries (Mays 1998), as the results from the site demonstrate. Moreover, the difference between the prevalence rate of caries for both sexes, males (12.7%) and females (27.1%), indicates a difference in diet and eating habits (Plate 15). Women were generally responsible for cooking and thus had more opportunity to snack on food (Ogden, pers. comm.).

Table 29 Dental pathology: number and percentage of teeth affected

	Male & Male?		Female & Female?		Adult*		Sub-adult deciduous	
	n	*%*	*n*	*%*	*n*	*%*	*n*	*%*
Total teeth	527	69.3	383	60.5	234	98.7	408	85.7
Postmortem loss	76	10	61	9.6	2	0.8	32	6.7
Antemortem loss	157	20.6	189	29.8	1	0.4	36	7.5
Caries	67	12.7	104	27.1	9	3.8	12	2.9
Abscesses	23	4.3	10	1.8	0	0	0	0
Calculus	270	51.2	87	22.7	0	0	13	3.1
Enamel hypoplasia	122	23.1	54	14	0	0	31	7.5

*Adult included indeterminate and sub-adult permanent teeth.

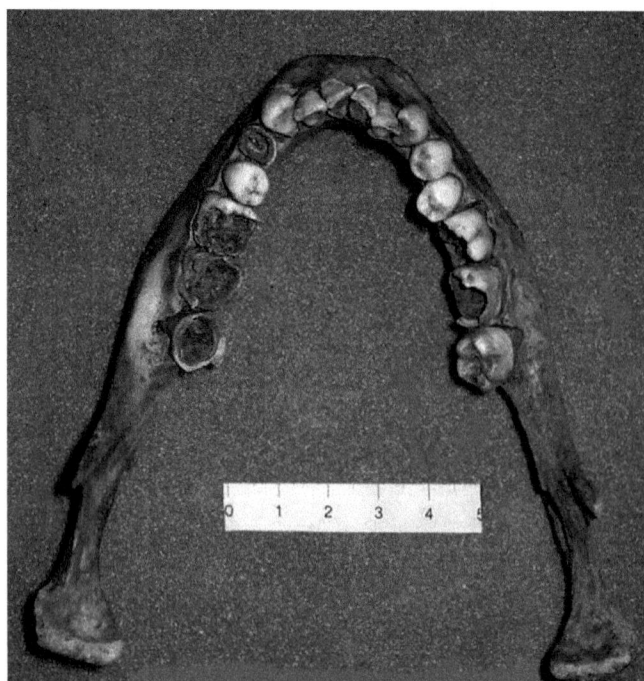

Plate 15 Occlusal caries from HB 53

Table 30 Numbers of permanent teeth with caries (both sides combined)

	Male		Female		Unsexed		Total
	max	man	max	man	max	man	
I1	0	2	6	6	0	0	14
I2	3	3	9	8	0	0	23
C	1	3	5	10	0	0	19
PM1	6	3	6	8	0	0	23
PM2	3	4	8	9	2	1	27
M1	6	7	6	5	2	1	27
M2	4	10	4	5	2	1	26
M3	5	7	4	5	0	0	21
Total	28	39	48	56	6	3	180

Table 31　　Caries – site frequency

Sex	Occlusal	Buccal	Lingual	Mesial	Distal	Multiple	Total
Male	13	14	1	19	11	12	70
Female	9	27	2	21	26	24	109
Indeterminate	0	0	1	0	0	0	1
Subadult	4	0	0	0	2	3	9
Total	26	41	4	40	39	39	189

Table 32 Number of deciduous teeth with caries (both sides combined)

	Sub-adult		Total
	max	man	
I1	2	0	2
I2	1	0	1
C	0	0	0
M1	2	1	3
M2	2	4	6
Total	7	5	12

Table 33 Caries (deciduous teeth) – site frequency

Age	Occlusal	Buccal	Lingual	Mesial	Distal	Multiple	Total
Subadult	3	0	1	2	4	2	12
Total	3	0	1	2	4	2	12

Caries were recorded according to the tooth and the site on which the cavity was positioned in the tooth (Tables 30 to 33). Caries were most commonly found on the second premolars and the first molars. However, caries can also lead to ante mortem tooth loss and, as the results in Table 28 show, first molars were the teeth most frequently lost ante mortem. Consequently, it is likely that the prevalence of caries in the first molars was higher than the initial results suggested. Finally, the distribution of the caries across the tooth revealed that all the tooth surfaces showed a similar prevalence rate of caries, with the exception of the lingual aspect, which was rarely affected by decay.

Abscesses
Located in the alveolar bone, abscesses are perforations of differing shapes and sizes caused by a collection of pus, originating at the apex of the root of a dead tooth.

Cysts and granulomas were recorded in the same category as abscesses, although they are a separate entity. Cysts had been considered to be chronic abscesses; however, presently they are described as a type of soft tissue tumour (Dias and Tayles 1997).

From this population, 33 skeletons showed abscesses (Table 34); none of them were in the juvenile category. Most abscesses were located in the maxillary area. This region is less robust than the mandible and consequently is more likely to be perforated. Furthermore, nearly 70% of abscesses were recorded in the male group. Comparing other skeletal populations from different time periods, it is possible to conclude that abscess prevalence at this site (2.8%) was higher than in Romano-British (1.2%) or Anglo-Saxon (0.7%) cemetery populations (Roberts and Cox 2003).

Table 34 Abscesses

Tooth position	Male		Female		Subadult		Total
	max	man	max	man	max	man	
I1	1	0	1	0	0	0	2
I2	1	0	0	0	0	0	1
C	2	0	0	0	0	0	2
PM1	1	0	1	0	0	0	2
PM2	2	2	1	1	0	0	6
M1	6	2	0	2	0	0	10
M2	3	3	2	0	0	0	8
M3	0	0	2	0	0	0	2
Total	16	7	7	3	0	0	33

Table 35 Calculus – teeth affected (both sides combined)

Tooth	Male & ? Male		Female & ? Female		Subadult		Total
	max	man	max	man	max	man	
I1	11	26	1	12	0	4	54
I2	13	28	3	13	1	2	60
C	16	29	3	11	1	0	60
PM1	14	26	2	9	2	0	53
PM2	12	21	1	8	1	0	43
M1	14	17	9	3	2	0	45
M2	13	12	6	1	0	0	32
M3	9	9	2	3	0	0	23
Total	102	168	27	60	7	6	370

Table 36 Enamel hypoplasia – teeth affected (both sides combined)

Tooth	Male		Female		Subadult		Total
	max	man	max	man	max	man	
I1	4	12	4	4	2	6	32
I2	5	14	6	9	2	6	42
C	16	34	3	13	4	6	76
PM1	7	20	0	6	0	0	33
PM2	4	6	0	3	1	0	14
M1	0	0	2	2	2	2	8
M2	0	0	2	0	0	0	2
M3	0	0	0	0	0	0	0
Total	36	86	17	37	11	20	207

Calculus

More commonly known as 'tartar', calculus is a hard deposit of mineralised plaque formed on the teeth and frequently attached to the surface next to the gums (Hillson 1996). It is a manifestation of the lack of dental hygiene in a skeletal population. At the site, half the male population manifested calculus, while only 22% of females did so and only 3% of juveniles were recorded with calculus (Table 35). As these results show, calculus rates increase with age. Another possible conclusion is that at this site females demonstrated more concern about dental hygiene than the male population.

Enamel hypoplasia

Dental enamel hypoplasia (DEH) is one of the most reliable stress indicators, occurring during childhood. Hypoplasia is a deficiency in the enamel thickness, caused by episodes of stress such as malnutrition, anaemia and high fever that affect the usual development of the enamel permanently (Hillson 1996). DEH was most often recorded in the mandibular canine, due to its developing later than other teeth (Table 36). Some 23% of males and 14% of females showed enamel hypoplasia in this collection, while only 7.5% of juveniles did so. One sole juvenile skeleton HB 125 (an adolescent probable male) showed an association between DEH and *cribra orbitalia*.

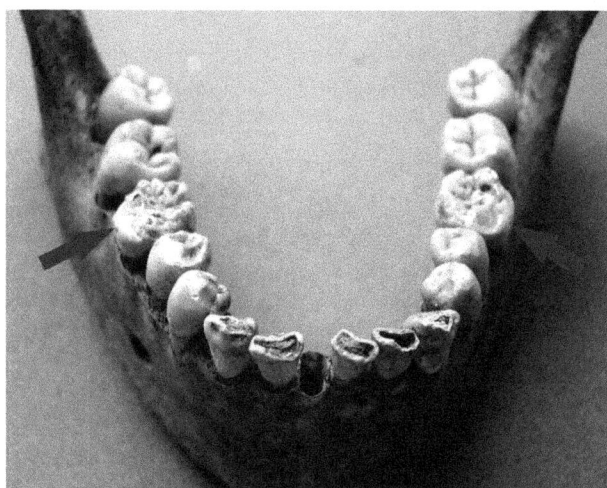

Plate 16 Dental enamel hypoplasia (arrows) from HB 70

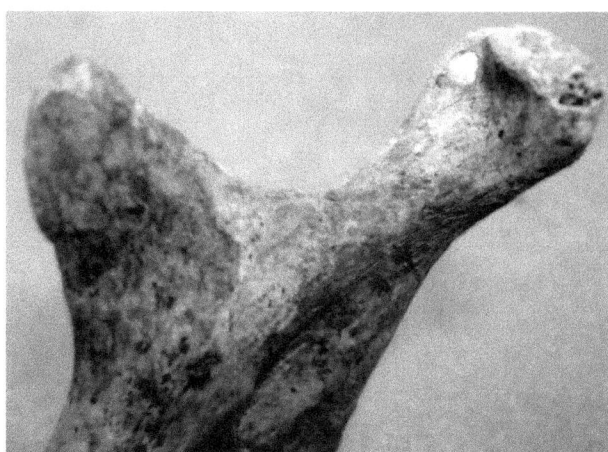

Plate 17 Tooth embedded in the condylar process of HB 75

One of the most severe cases of DEH was HB 70, a male whose identity is known. The particular appearance of all four first molars may be related to the severity of DEH, which interrupted the normal development of the cusps and suggests that this individual had suffered an episode of severe malnutrition or high fever between birth and six months of age (Ogden, pers. comm.) (Plate 16). HB 70 was identified from the legible *depositum* plate associated with the burial as James White, who died in 1827 at the age of 42. A trade directory reveals that he was a grocer and a tea dealer (see Chapter 6).

The prevalence of the enamel hypoplasia was similar to that found at other contemporary sites like the Redcross Way burials (Brickley and Miles 1999). This in itself is intriguing as Redcross Way was a pauper burial ground. However the prevalence was high compared with Spitalfields, a wealthier group from the same time period (Molleson *et al* 1993), and much lower than the prevalence recorded from excavations at St Martin's in Birmingham (69%) (Brickley *et al* 2006). However, recording methods differed between these studies.

Periodontal disease
This pathology results from chronic infection of the gingival soft tissues, leading to chronic periodontitis and to destruction of alveolar bone. As a consequence, it causes exposure of the root tooth or, in the most extreme cases, loss of the tooth. Various factors initiate the pathological process like calculus and metabolic bone disease (Brickley and Miles 1999).

The scoring of severity in periodontal disease is sometimes problematic because the recession of alveolar bone can be confused with compensatory eruption of the teeth, which happens due to ageing or attrition. In this study the scoring system of different degree of severity was based on Ogden's (unpublished) methodology (Appendix 1). A total of 18 individuals from the site were affected by periodontal disease. However, these figures could be an underestimate because it is impossible to

identify the first stage of the disease (which is seen in the soft tissues) and the last stage (when the skeleton becomes toothless). Males illustrated more prevalence of periodontal disease than females. Furthermore, the most severe cases were in the mature adult category (46+).

Dental anomalies
Most of the dental anomalies present in this skeletal assemblage are related to the number of teeth, their position on the jaws, and eruption. In some individuals the third molars were absent, due to a congenital abnormality. In others, deciduous teeth or roots were retained, pushing the permanent teeth lingually or palatally. A canine (HB104), for instance, was unerupted, being retained under the palatine bone. HB 56, a middle-aged male, showed various dental anomalies: a strange crown shape of the upper left M3, retention of a deciduous root, as well as root disruption to the maxillary incisors and canines, perhaps due to a childhood fracture.

Carabelli's cusps, a minor variant used as a non-metric trait, were recorded in two individuals. In one of these (HB 75), a possible right M3 was located under the condylar process of the mandible (Plate 17). There was an oro-antral fistula (HB 93) with a large bony exostosis containing the roots of the upper left M2 on the floor of the maxillary antrum, which was related to the fistula. Finally, a more unusual anomaly traced in just one skeleton (HB 28) was an enamel pearl on the mesial root.

Dental wear
Dental wear was not used as an age-at-death determination method, since it is not very reliable as an age indicator for this period. Nevertheless, in some individuals wear patterns were recorded in order to determine the presence of pipe smokers. Three individuals (HB 96, 99 and 130), all of them old middle adult males, had a semicircular abrasion from a stem pipe on the maxillary and mandibular canines, PM1 or second incisor of both sides (Plate 18).

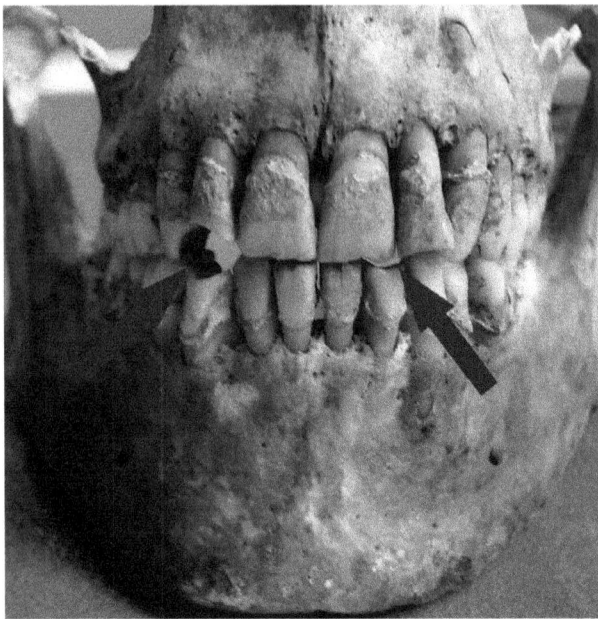

Plate 18 Dental wear from pipe-smoking in HB 96

Skeletal pathology

The analysis for bone changes and pathology was performed on the skeletal assemblage from the site in order to gain a better understanding of health and disease in 19th-century Wolverhampton. This is of particular importance when comparing how living conditions affected archaeological populations from different periods and environments.

Trauma

The study of fractures, injuries and dislocations provides an indicator of lifestyle and occupation, and evidence of interpersonal violence (Roberts and Manchester 1995).

Fractures

Tables 37 and 38 depict the number of fractures according to the most frequent site on the skeleton. The highest number of fractures was evident in both sexes on the ribs, followed by the hands. However, the most notable fractures were those to the face and bones of the upper limb. There had been severe trauma to the left proximal humerus of HB 75 (Plate 20), a female who was also suffering from syphilis. Both first metacarpals and the left fourth metacarpal of HB 120, a male, showed healed fractures with some crushing of the hand bones involved. These injuries are suggestive of accidents at work or, in the case of HB 120 who also had fractured nasal bones, a sport like boxing. Another male, HB 40 (Plate 19), had fractured both nasal bones and had healed fractures around the entire left orbital area, possibly due to boxing. A depressed fracture was found in the left parietal of HB 46.

Unhealed, or perimortem, fractures were found in the right humerus and right femur of HB 44, a male who was suffering from syphilis. The reason for his violent death is open to question but the site of the fractures might suggest a fall from a great height.

A compression fracture was found in HB 15 on the right side of the vertebral body of T12 and L1, which in turn had resulted in the fusion of the two vertebrae and lateral deviation (scoliosis) of that area of the spine.

Table 37   Fractures in the male sample

Bone	Male and Male?					
	Right	%	Left	%	Unsided	%
Clavicle	0/17	0	1/20	5	0	0
Humerus	0/29	0	0/24	0	0	0
Radius	0/28	0	1/22	4.5	0	0
Ulna	0/31	0	0/23	0	0	0
Hand (metacarpals)	3/30	10	2/25	8	0	0
Ribs	1/27	3.7	3/28	10.7	5/28	17.8
Femur	1/27	3.7	0/24	0	0	0

Table 38 Fractures in the female sample

Bone	Female and Female?					
	Right	%	Left	%	Unsided	%
Clavicle	0/22	0	0/17	0	0	0
Humerus	0/25	0	2/26	7.6	0	0
Radius	0/22	0	0/21	0	0	0
Ulna	1/24	4.1	0/25	0	0	0
Hand (metacarpals)	1/25	4	0/25	0	0	0
Ribs	2/31	6.4	0/31	0	7/31	22.5
Femur	0/24	0	0/27	0	0	0

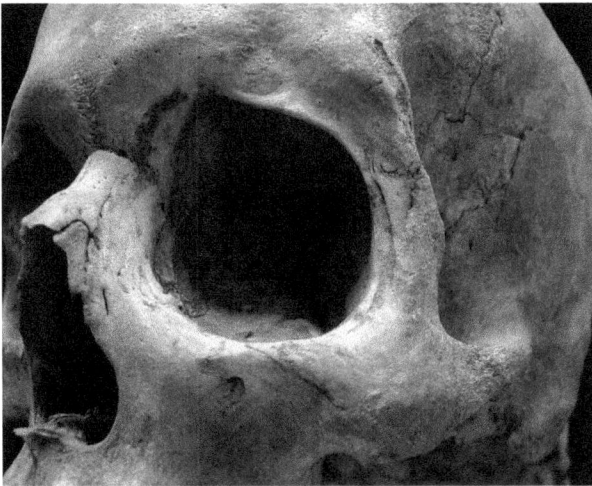

Plate 19 Fractured nasal bone and orbital rim of HB 40

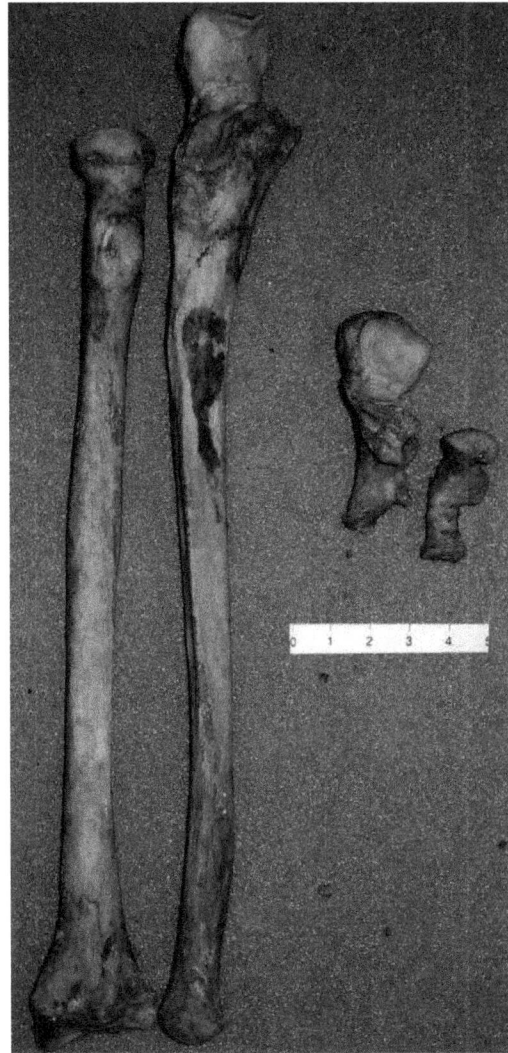

Plate 21 Left arm amputation from HB 53

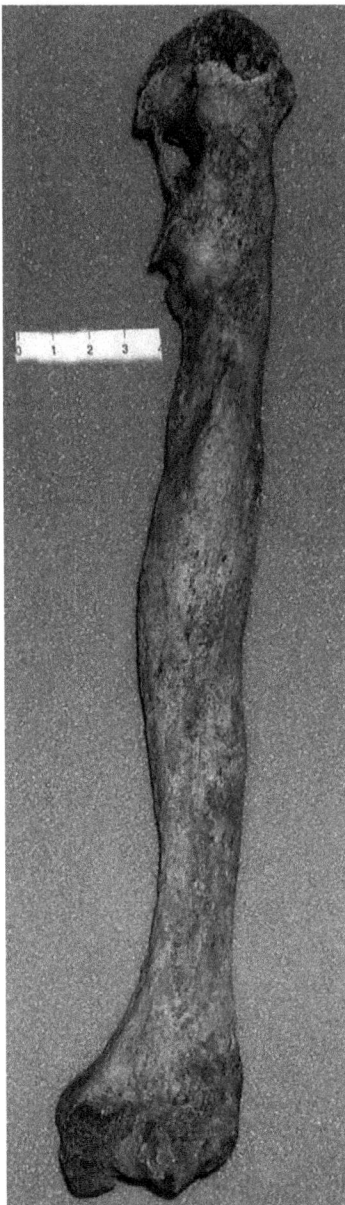

Plate 20 Fracture of humerus in HB 75

Amputations

Three cases of amputation (HB 53, HB 86 and HB 129) were found. The first individual (Plate 21) had had her left arm amputated just below the elbow (left radius and ulna). The forearm bones were represented by stubs which suggested a traumatic event such as catching the arm in a machine (Manchester, pers. comm.) The second case (Plate 22) had an amputation of the left tibia and fibula. The third (Plate 23) had an amputation of the right femur. There was a healed femoral neck fracture in the same bone. Whether the amputations were carried out as the result of disease or an accident remains unresolved. Nevertheless, it is certain that whatever the cause of such traumatic incidents, at least in HB 53 and HB 129, amputation took place long before death. These two examples show clear evidence of well-healed amputations and disuse atrophy of the amputated limbs.

Myositis ossificans traumatica

One of the lesions occurring on the bone that can represent prior damage to the muscle is *myositis ossificans traumatica* (Plate 24). Depending on how

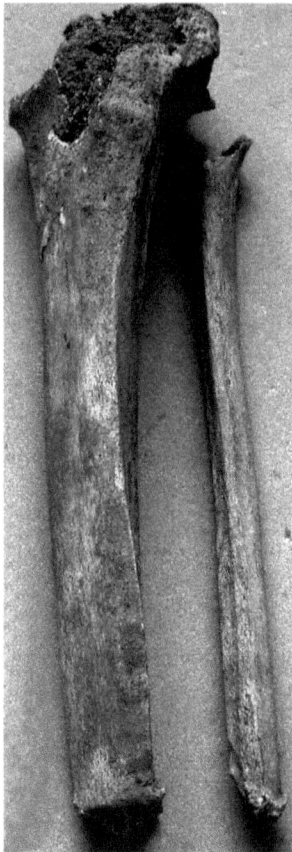

Plate 22 Amputation of tibia and fibula in HB 86

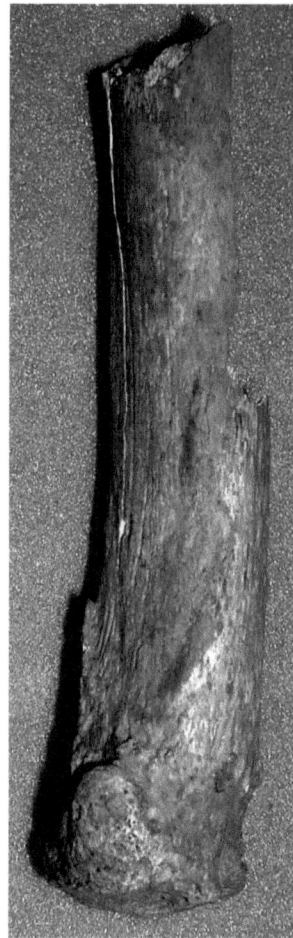

Plate 23 Amputated right femur from HB 129

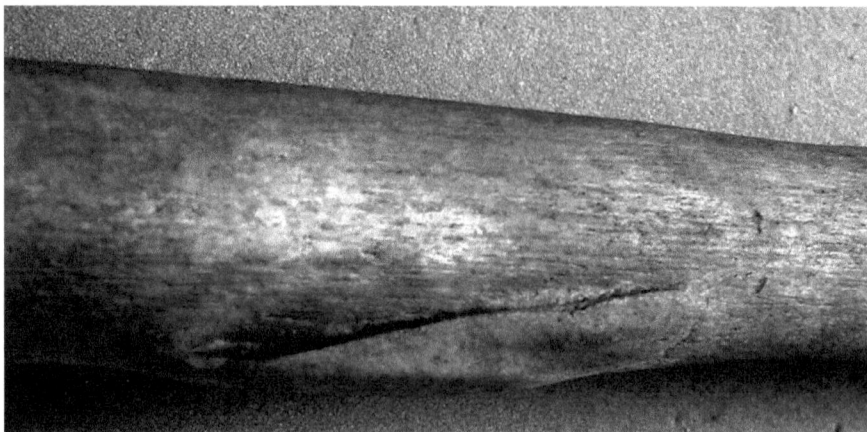

Plate 24 *Myositis ossificans traumatica* in HB 146

severe the injury is, the muscle sometimes responds by producing bone in the muscle tissue itself (Ortner 2003). This was the case in seven individuals from the site, of whom five (HB 92, 96, 99, 146 and 148) suffered from this condition in their femora and another two individuals (HB 75 and 124) in their humeri, with differing degrees of severity.

Osteochondritis dissecans

This is the result of local trauma where a piece of bone detaches itself from the joint surface as consequence of trauma and the death of the cartilage and/ or a circulatory disorder of the joint (Roberts and Cox 2003). Three individuals had suffered this condition on the humeral surface of the elbow joint: HB 19, HB 40 (Plate 25) and HB 89 and only one individual (HB 76) on both condyles of the right femur.

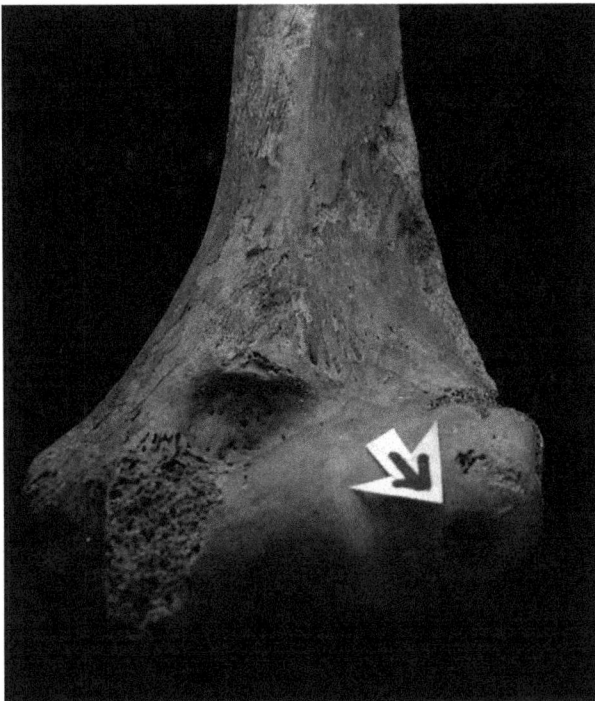

Plate 25 *Osteochondritis dissecans* in HB 40

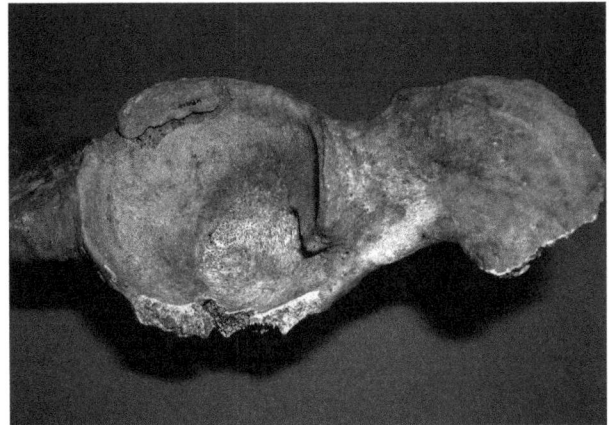

Plate 26 Developmental defects on left acetabular rim of HB 44

Congenital abnormalities

Congenital abnormalities are often called developmental abnormalities and are the result of problems during embryological development. One of the commonest conditions is *spina bifida occulta* in which the neural arches of one or more vertebrae fail to develop, although this is of minor or no clinical significance (Ortner 2003). This was the case in one woman (HB 28) who had complete *spina bifida* of the sacrum.

Other conditions occurring during development without adverse consequences or symptomatology are the cranio-caudal shifts that take place during the segmentation of the spine. Generally, this process occurs at the borders between spinal areas (eg the cervico-thoracic junction), resulting in segmental disarrangement and sometimes producing rudimentary unilateral or bilateral supernumerary ribs. For instance, HB 128 had a fragment of cervical vertebra with a costal facet for a cervical rib and the tenth thoracic vertebrae had a costal facet on the right transverse process and none on the left. A similar

example was found in HB 70 where the seventh cervical vertebrate had two costal facets (one on the body and other on the transverse process to articulate with a small cervical rib) but only on the left-hand side.

An unusual case that could have been the product of a developmental defect is HB 44 (Plate 26). An ossicle of trapezoidal shape measuring 28mm in length by 11mm in width was found disarticulated from the left acetabular rim. Furthermore, the auricular surface of the joint between sacrum and pelvic bone had a deep concavity, which could also have been the product of a developmental anomaly. The right tympanic plate of the right temporal bone of HB 99 was incomplete and the external auditory meatus was considerably larger than the left.

Non-specific infection

A number of bacteria are responsible for producing non-specific infections (Roberts and Cox 2003). Periostitis, osteitis and osteomyelitis are types of non-specific infection. Periostitis is also termed 'periosteal reaction' and produces superficial inflammation and new bone deposits. Osteitis is the inflammation of the cortical bone and osteomyelitis indicates inflammation of the entire bone including the marrow cavity. Although they may have not been the direct cause of death, infectious diseases affecting the skeleton are chronic and longstanding.

Table 39   Males and females affected by non-specific infection

Site of Infection	Male and Male?				Female and Female?			
	Right	%	Left	%	Right	%	Left	%
Humerus	2/29	6.8	2/24	8.3	1/25	4	1/26	3.8
Radius	2/28	7.1	1/22	4.5	0/19	0	0/19	0
Ulna	2/31	6.4	1/23	4.3	0/24	0	0/25	0
Femur	3/27	11.1	1/24	4.1	3/24	12.5	3/27	11.1
Tibia	2/17	11.7	5/19	26.3	1/15	6.6	3/17	17.6
Fibula	3/8	37.5	3/9	33.3	3/6	50	1/6	16.6

Table 40 Indeterminate individuals affected by non-specific infection

Site of infection	Indeterminate sex			
	Right	%	Left	%
Humerus	0/1	0	0/1	0
Radius	0/1	0	0/2	0
Ulna	0/2	0	0/3	0
Femur	0/3	0	0/0	0
Tibia	3/5	60	2/2	100
Fibula	2/5	40	2/4	50

Periostitis
The most common sites of infection were the tibia and fibula (Table 39). It was notable that periosteal reactions in these two bones were considerably more frequent in males than in females. Individuals of indeterminate sex (Table 40) had more periostitis on the tibiae than the fibulae.

Maxillary sinusitis
Maxillary sinusitis is caused by an inflammation of the nasal mucosa that expands to the antral mucosa exposing it to bacterial attack and therefore to sinusitis (Boocock *et al* 1995). Nowadays it is associated with poor air quality and pollution, allergies and infections of the upper respiratory tract (Lewis *et al* 1995). Infection can also spread from dental disease (eg abscesses) and produce sinusitis, in which case it can make the distinction difficult. Where the cranium was complete, it was impossible to observe the sinuses. However, it was possible to determine that one male (HB 99), one female (HB 104) and one indeterminate individual (HB 82) had infective changes in one or both of their sinus cavities.

Rib lesions
Evidence of inflammatory processes on the visceral surfaces of the ribs is quite common in archaeological material (Plate 27). In fact, deposition of new bone formation can occur several times during the life of a person (Roberts *et al* 1998). There is general agreement in considering rib lesions to be the result of pulmonary infection that produced an inflammatory reaction on the visceral surface of the ribs. However, for the rib to be affected by a pulmonary infection (specific or non-specific) and develop periostitis, the disease needs to be a chronic and long-standing one such as tuberculosis. In the St Peter's sample both sexes had rib lesions predominantly on the left-hand side of the rib cage (Table 41). Women in particular were slightly more affected than men.

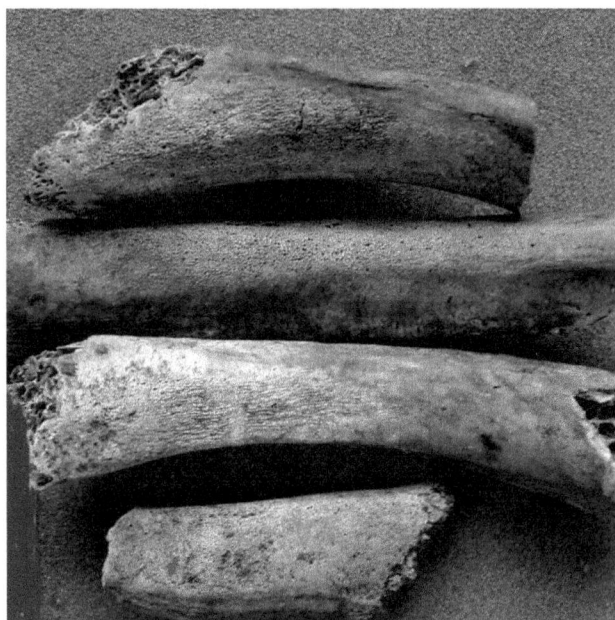

Plate 27 Rib lesions in HB 119

Cranium
Periosteal reactions are very common lesions encountered on the cranial vault bones, particularly in young infants. The cause of these lesions is difficult to ascertain. In the St Peter's population, six young children displayed deposits of porous and woven new bone formation on either the inner or outer table of the skull (Table 42). A young adult female (HB 119) has porous lesions scattered in several areas of the cranium, including the glabella region, around the sagittal suture, on both parietals, near the external occipital protuberance, on both orbits and both zygomatic bones and on both maxillae.

Specific infection
Specific infections, where the causative organism is known, include tuberculosis, leprosy and syphilis. There were two possible cases of syphilis and one of tuberculosis. The first one (HB 44) showed evidence of chronic infection in the right tibia. This was swollen and completely remodelled. HB 75 demonstrated syphilitic lesions with sclerosing osteomyelitis and periostitis on the right tibia and fibula. Both bones showed severe remodelling.

Only one case (HB 40) had lytic lesions in the spine compatible with tuberculosis (Plate 28). Two lumbar vertebrae showed destruction of the anterior portion of their bodies by almost 75% (Lumbar 1) and 95%

Table 41 Number of males and females affected by rib lesions

Male and Male? (Rib lesion)				Female and Female? (Rib lesion)			
Right	%	Left	%	Right	%	Left	%
4/27	14.8	5/28	17.8	4/31	12.9	6/31	19.3

Table 42 Individuals with cranial evidence of non-specific infection

Skeleton	Age	Area of the cranium
HB64	0-3 months	Deposits of woven bone on the inner and outer table of the occipital, both parietals and a fragment of frontal. Both orbital roofs affected similarly.
HB100	6-8 months	Deposits of porous new bone formation on the outer and inner surfaces of temporal bones.
HB132	6 months-1year	Deposits of woven bone on the inner table of one probable fragment of parietal.
HB102	1-2 years	Deposits of localised new bone formation on temporal bones and on both mandibular fossae.
HB24	<2years	Deposits of woven and porous new bone on 9 (inner and outer table) fragments of parietal.
HB82	14-18 years	Deposits of porous new bone formation on the outer surface of both greater wings of the sphenoids.

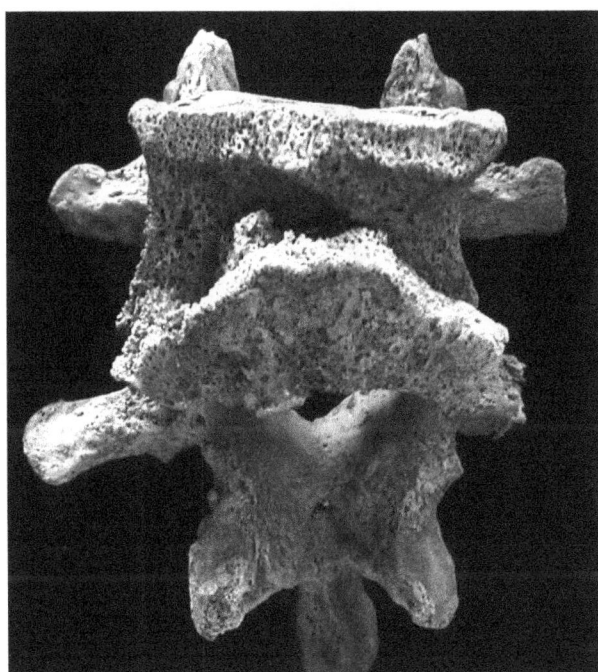

Plate 28 Tuberculosis. Lytic lesions on spine of HB 40

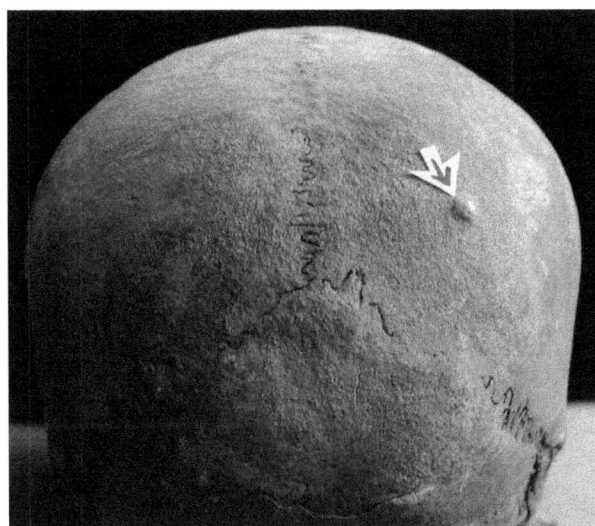

Plate 29 Osteoma from HB 112

(Lumbar 2). The lytic lesions have produced cavitation of the bodies, which in turn led to the collapse of the L1 on L2. The two vertebrae are fused through their apophyseal joints and their neural arches are preserved. These bone changes are characteristic of tuberculosis.

Metabolic diseases
In the archaeological record, metabolic diseases are associated with nutritional problems as a result of either an excess or a deficiency of a specific food component (Ortner 2003). Metabolic diseases encompass a wide range of conditions such as rickets, *cribra orbitalia*, scurvy, osteoporosis and Harris lines. Only the first three of these were identified from individuals from the site.

Rickets
This is a skeletal deformation caused by a deficiency in vitamin D that affects children in their early years (Aufderheide and Rodríguez-Martín 1998). Vitamin D plays an important role in the mineralisation of bone and therefore its lack during growth affects the ability of the weight-bearing bones to support biomechanical stress, leading to deformity (Ortner 2003). Exposing skin to light can compensate for the lack of vitamin D intake. However, the urban areas of England that were growing as a consequence of 17th- and 18th-century industrialisation produced environments (smoke-filled air and high population density) that prevented skin from synthesising and absorbing vitamin D.

One of the characteristics of rickets is the medio-lateral bowing of the upper and lower limbs (although an antero-posterior bowing can also occur). Only four infants from the site demonstrated evidence of rickets (HB 30, 52, 102 and 106). The first infant showed an abnormal flaring of the upper metaphysis of the right humerus and the same pattern on three right ribs (Plate 32). The second infant

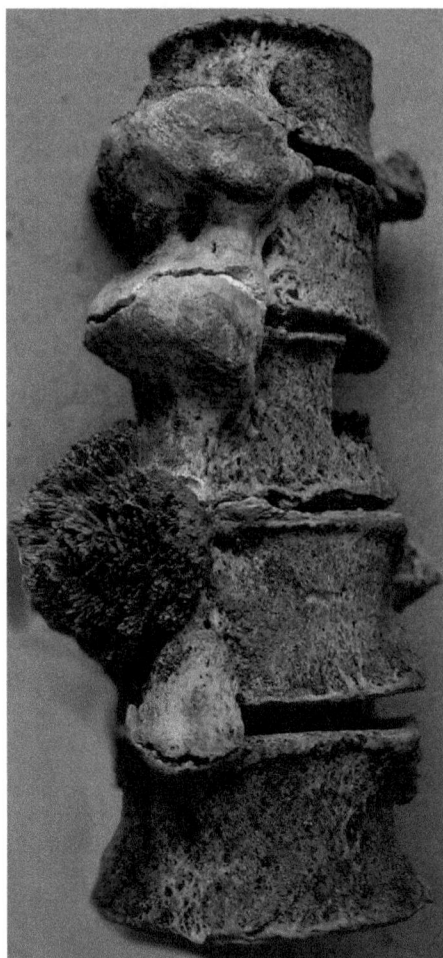

Plate 30 Primary neoplasm from HB 39

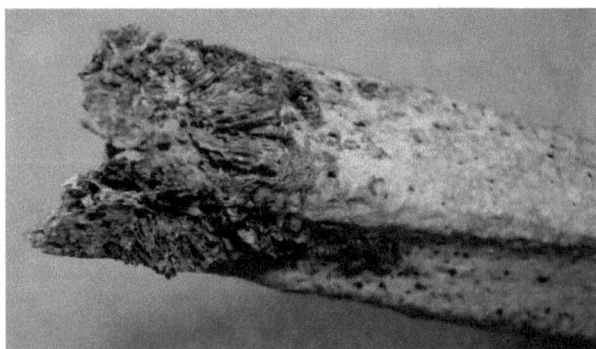

Plate 31 'Sunburst' lesion on ribs found with context HB 40

had medio-lateral bowing of both tibiae and fibulae. Two young children, HB 102 and HB 106, had antero-posterior bowing of the left femur (the former) and a medio-lateral bowing of both fibulae (the latter).

Deficiency of vitamin D acquired in adulthood is called osteomalacia (Aufderheide and Rodríguez-Martín 1998). HB 70 (identified as James White) was the only adult male individual with evidence of bowing in both radii, ulnae and fibulae (Plate 33). This is probably as a consequence of inadequate intake of vitamin D during early childhood (rickets) or during adulthood

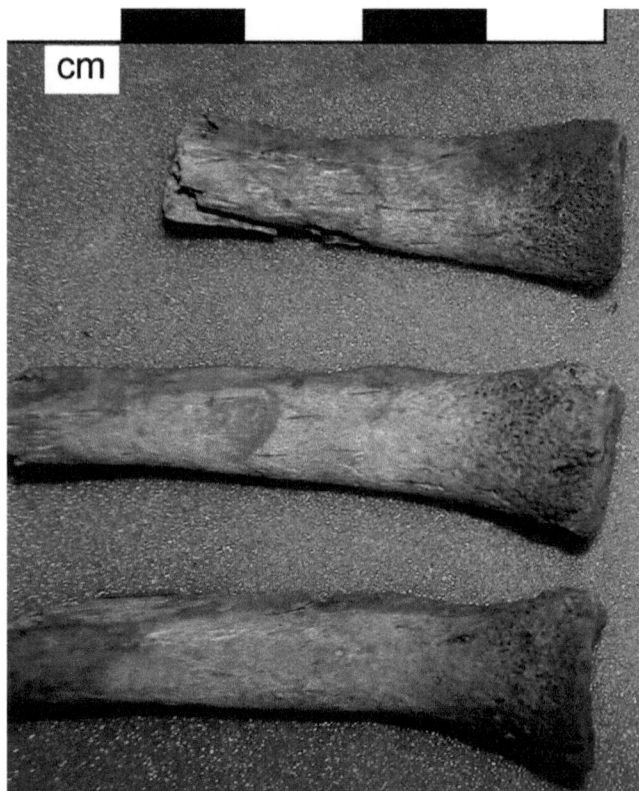

Plate 32 Evidence for rickets (abnormal flaring of rib ends) in HB 52

(osteomalacia) as demonstrated by abnormal remodelling of the bone matrix. His severe enamel hypoplasia suggests that rickets occurred in infancy, ie during the first year of life.

Cribra orbitalia

This is a sieve-like lesion located on the orbital roofs (Plate 34). Although its cause remains obscure, most writers support the association of *cribra orbitalia* and iron deficiency anaemia (Stuart-Macadam 1987, 1991, 1992). It is highly valuable as a stress marker to assess how populations adapted to a particular environment in the past (Boylston and Roberts 2004). The severity and location of the lesions was graded according to Stuart-Macadam's (1991) technique. *Cribra orbitalia* was very common in the juvenile population from the site, affecting both orbits in 24.1% of children (Table 43). Severity was moderate (type 2 and type 3) in nine orbital roofs and most often located on the antero-lateral (31.2%), antero-intermediate (37.5%) and antero-medial (31.2%) sector of the orbits.

Scurvy

Scurvy is produced by prolonged deficiency in vitamin C intake. The ascorbic acid contained in vitamin C is responsible for collagen formation in the bone. Therefore, its absence during the first stages of life produces poor bone matrix, which in turn leads to skeletal growth retardation and irreversible skeletal changes. For instance, subperiosteal haemorrhages due to chronic bleeding are among the commonest features (Ortner

Table 43   Comparison of number of cases with *cribra orbitalia*

Orbit	Male	%	Female	%	Sub-adult	%
Right	1/25	4	0/26	0	7/29	24.1
Left	1/26	3.8	0/26	0	7/29	24.1

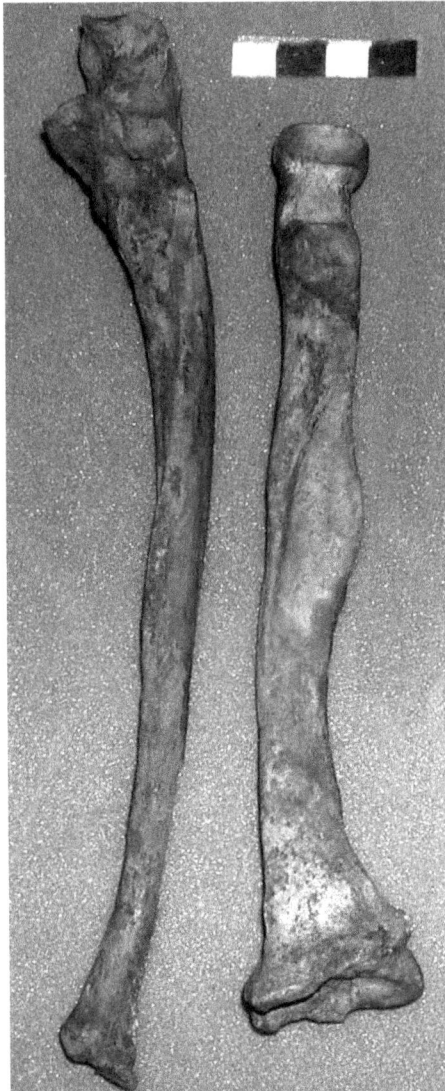

Plate 33 Bowing of radius and ulna from HB 70 (vitamin D deficiency)

2003). The skeletal diagnosis consists of evidence of new bone formation in areas where soft tissues have been associated with traumatised blood vessels (Roberts and Cox 2003). One individual from the site (HB 103) appeared to have been suffering from this condition. The child exhibited widespread porous bone deposits on both orbital roofs. A fragment of cranial vault also showed deposits of new bone on the endocranial surface. These pathological changes can be indicative of this kind of nutritional deficiency.

Neoplasia

The term neoplasm refers to 'new tissue' or 'mass of new tissue'. Neoplastic tissue can be malignant or benign depending on whether its proliferation is capable of destroying surrounding cells or not (Aufderheide and Rodríguez-Martín 1998). One of the commonest benign tumours found in archaeological specimens is the so-called osteoma, button osteoma, spongy exostosis or ivory exostosis (Plate 29), generally of nodular shape and composed of hard dense bone. From the site, a total of three cases of cranial osteoma were found. Two of them (HB 112 and 143) had solitary osteomas located on the posterior side of the left and right parietal respectively. On the other hand, HB 36 had four osteomas located on the frontal bone.

An elderly female (HB 124) had multiple rounded and protruding bony formations scattered in several regions of the skull, such as the right zygomatic process of the supraorbital margin, and also in the region of glabella. In the occipital bone, they are present along the nuchal crest and external occipital protuberance. They are also found at both asterions and on the tuberosity of the left maxilla. The mandible was affected in a similar manner with a bony formation or exostosis at the site of the right M3 socket. Ortner (2003) describes a case of multiple osteoblastic lesions present in several areas of the skull and particularly accentuated on the occipital bone that resembles the cranial exostoses present on HB 124 (Plate 35). According to Ortner, this could be a benign fibro-osseous tumour.

Malignant tumours

Malignant tumours are rarely found in Britain before the post-medieval period. Three cases of malignant tumour were found in individuals from the site. A striking case of primary neoplasm was found in an elderly male (HB 39), which showed exuberant 'sunbursts' of bone of 33mm in diameter and 32mm in height on the anterior right-hand side of the tenth and eleventh vertebral bodies (Plate 30). This pattern was also present on the visceral side of one mid-thoracic left rib and the shaft of an unidentified rib. In both cases the pattern extends perpendicular to the surface of the bone. Six other ribs from the left-hand side and six from the right side were also affected but not so dramatically. The general condition of the skeleton was very porous and friable with multiple perforated lesions which had rounded and sharp margins spread all over the bony surfaces. These lesions were present on the inner and outer table of the skull, spine, sacrum and both os coxae. The most likely diagnosis for this tumour is osteosarcoma.

Some of the additional material associated with HB 40 was composed of two fragmentary right ribs (one middle and the other lower thoracic) and one head fragment from

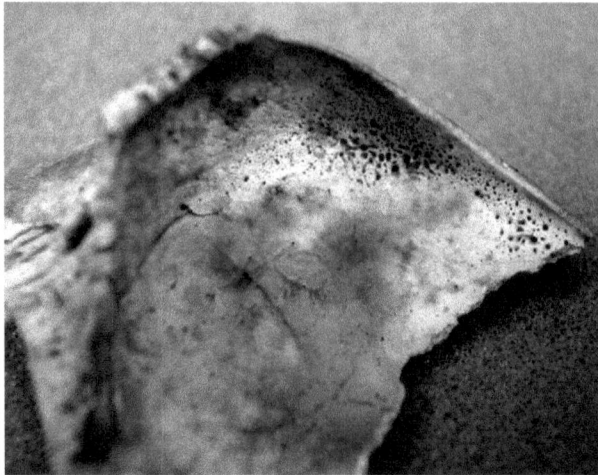

Plate 34 *Cribra orbitalia* in HB 106

the left upper ribs (Plate 31). There were also three unidentified rib shaft fragments. All these ribs had multiple perforated lesions ranging from 0.5mm to 3mm with rounded and sharp margins. Two of the above were associated with new bone formation or 'sunbursts' of bone extending perpendicular to the surface of the bone on the visceral side of the ribs. These pathological changes are compatible with metastases from a primary neoplasm whose site is unclear.

The axial skeleton of a middle-aged male (HB 84) displayed dispersed lytic lesions with sharp margins in the vertebral bodies, ribs and os coxae. Rounded and lytic lesions were also found in the mid shaft of two right-hand side ribs. These pathological changes found on the skeleton may represent a widespread malignant secondary carcinoma or multiple myeloma.

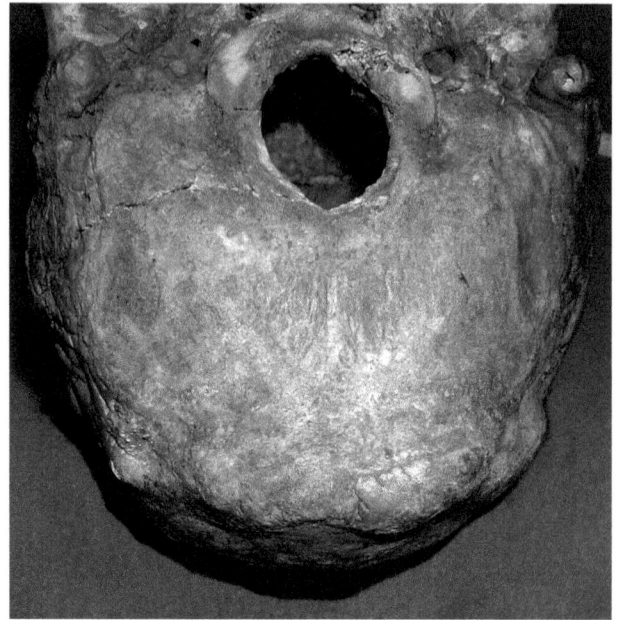

Plate 35 Cranial exostoses from HB 124

Joint disease

One of the most common pathological conditions present in archaeological material is joint disease or osteoarthritis (OA). The skeletal assemblage from the site was diagnosed for osteoarthritis according to the methodology of Rogers and Waldron (1995). This multifactorial and worldwide condition affects the synovial joints of the axial and appendicular skeleton (Rogers and Waldron 1995; Larsen 1997). Population studies have found that age, sex, genetic predisposition, hormonal influence, nutrition, mechanical stress, trauma, environmental conditions and physical activity are variables associated with the disorder (Rogers and Waldron 1995; Jurmain

Table 44   Number of individuals affected by OA

Joint	Male and Male?				Female and Female?			
	Right	%	Left	%	Right	%	Left	%
Temporo-mandibular	1/26	4	0/26	0	0/27	0	0/27	0
Gleno-humeral	2/22	9	2/25	8	0/22	0	1/23	4.3
Acromio-clavicular	4/17	23.5	3/20	15	0/19	0	1/16	6.2
Elbow	1/29	3.4	1/24	4.1	2/25	8	1/26	3.8
Hand*	5/30	16.6	4/25	16	4/25	16	4/25	16
Costo-clavicular	0/27	0	1/27	3.7	0/27	0	0/27	0
Costo-manubrial	0/27	0	0/27	0	0/27	0	1/27	3.7
Costo-vertebral	0/27	0	0/27	0	4/27	14.8	0/27	0
Hip	0/28	0	1/21	4.7	0/20	0	0/22	0
Knee	0/23	0	0/21	0	1/17	5.8	0/21	0
Foot*	4/14	29	1/14	7.1	2/14	14.2	0/12	0

*one or more joints

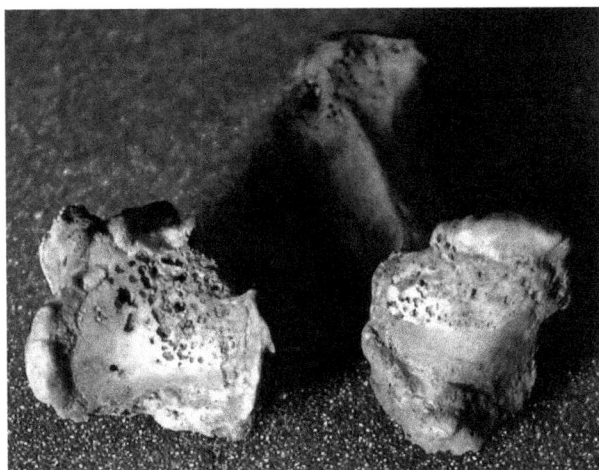

Plate 36 Evidence for OA in the hand bones of HB 23

1999; Roberts and Cox 2003). Despite the controversy surrounding the linkage between OA and activity, there is general agreement among bioarchaeologists that it may be a good indicator of activities carried out by human populations in the past (Jurmain 1999; Larsen 1997). Physically demanding lifestyles and strenuous labour result in injuries to the joints, thus increasing the risk of developing OA.

Synovial joints
Table 44 shows the number of individuals affected by OA in the synovial joints. Comparison between the sexes showed that men were severely affected by OA in both feet. In the female group the hands showed the highest percentages of OA, in one or more synovial joints (Plate 36).

Table 45   OA of spine in males

M and M?	Cervical	Thoracic	Lumbar
HB36	C1-C3	T1, T4-T8, T10	L4-L5
HB43	-	T8-T10	-
HB46	-	T3-T4, T6	-
HB54	-	T1, T11	-
HB85	C1, C4	-	-
HB93	-	T6	-
HB129	C1-C2	-	-
HB130	C1-C2	-	-
HB143	C1-C4, C7	-	-

Spinal joint disease
OA of the spine is generally present on the apophyseal joints of the vertebrae. Differences between males and females were very marked (p<0.001), as seen in Tables 45 and 46. Major dissimilarities were found in the thoracic area where males were more affected than females. In the lumbar spine women were more affected by far than men with the involvement of L2–L5. Only one man had OA of the lower back, from L4–L5. This difference may be indicating that women suffered from

significant stress on the lower spine compared with the thoracic spine in men, possibly associated with pregnancy.

Table 46 OA of spine in females

F and F?	Cervical	Thoracic	Lumbar
HB2	-	T3, T5	-
HB15	-	T12	L3, L5
HB37	C4	T2	L2-L4
HB47	C1-C2	-	-
HB67	-	T9	-
HB76	C3-C5	T12	L3-L4
HB90	C2	-	L5
HB104	C2, C5	T10-T11	-
HB109	C3-C5	-	-
HB124	-	T4	-
HB128	-	T4-T5, T10	-

Table 47   Number of individuals with spinal osteophytosis

Vertebra	M and M?	%	F and F?	%
C1	8/24	33.3	8/25	32.0
C2	9/25	36.0	5/21	23.8
C3	2/22	9.0	1/21	4.7
C4	4/22	18.1	3/23	13.0
C5	6/22	27.2	2/21	9.5
C6	4/21	19.0	7/22	31.8
C7	4/22	18.1	4/19	21.0
T1	3/21	14.2	2/20	10
T2	2/19	10.5	2/22	9.0
T3	0/19	0	1/22	4.5
T4	2/19	10.5	4/22	18.1
T5	0/17	0	6/22	27.2
T6	4/18	22.2	6/22	27.2
T7	3/18	16.6	4/21	19.0
T8	4/19	21.0	3/21	14.2
T9	5/17	29.4	6/21	28.5
T10	6/17	35.2	4/22	18.1
T11	7/19	36.8	4/21	19.0
T12	6/21	28.5	3/19	15.7
L1	4/22	18.1	2/21	9.5
L2	6/24	28.5	2/23	8.6
L3	7/23	30.4	1/23	4.3
L4	3/18	16.6	2/23	8.6
L5	4/19	21.0	2/21	9.5

Osteophytosis
Osteophytes are fringes of new bone that form at the margins of the vertebral bodies and around joint areas (Brickley and Miles 1999). Marginal osteophytosis on the upper and lower vertebral bodies was very common in the skeletons recovered from the site (Table 47). Females showed high rates of vertebral osteophytosis on two cervical vertebrae (C6–C7) and in the thoracic spine from T3 to T7. High percentages were also found in the first two cervical vertebrae (C1 and C2) of both sexes.

Table 48 Comparison between synovial and spinal joints in men and women

M & M?	Temp/mand.	Gleno/hum.	Acrom/clavic.	Elbow	Hand	Costo/vert.	Hip	Knee	Foot	Cervical	Thoracic	Lumbar
HB36		R/L	R/L		R/L		L		R	C1-C3	T1, T4-T8, T10	L4-L5
HB43											T8-T10	
HB46											T3-T4, T6	
HB54			R		R						T1, T11	
HB70				L								
HB85										C1, C4		
HB92		R										
HB93	R	L									T6	
HB108			L		L							
HB129			R		R/L					C1-C2		
HB130					R/L				R/L	C1-C2		
HB143			R/L							C1-C4, C7		
HB146				R								
F & F?												
HB2											T3, T5	
HB15											T12	L3, L5
HB23					R/L							
HB37					L					C4	T2	L2-L4
HB47										C1-C2		
HB67						R					T9	
HB76		L	L					R		C3-C5	T12	L3-L4
HB90										C2		L5
HB91									R			
HB98					R/L	R						
HB104										C2, C5	T10-T11	
HB109										C3-C5		
HB111									R			
HB124				R/L		R					T4	
HB128											T4-T5, T10	

Synovial and spinal joints affected with OA
When synovial joints of the spine are compared with those of the appendicular skeleton, it is evident that seven out of 14 male individuals had OA in both regions of the skeleton. The other half had OA in either one or another region (three of them in the axial skeleton and four in the appendicular). Five females had OA in both areas compared with eleven who suffered from the condition in either one or the other region (seven of them were affected in the axial skeleton and the four remaining in the appendicular skeleton).

From the site, 16 females out of 41 (females and probable females) and 14 males out of 39 (males and probable males) suffered from OA, which corresponds to 39.0% and 35.9% in each category respectively (Table 48).

Spondyloarthropathies
This is a generic term that refers to a group of arthropathies (disease or abnormality of the joints) that share several features in common, such as the involvement of the axial joints (spine or sacro-iliac joints) producing either erosion or fusion (Rothschild and Woods 1991). Elderly male HB 85 showed evidence of suffering from one of the seronegative spondyloarthropathies. Two pairs of cervical vertebrae were ankylosed through their right-hand side articular processes. Also elderly woman HB 149 had two unsided ribs fused to vertebral fragments through the tubercle. This might suggest ankylosing spondylitis. In the spine two mid-thoracic vertebrae and three lower thoracic vertebrae were fused through their apophyseal joints, suggesting an erosive arthropathy.

Activity-induced pathology
Determining what occupations past populations practised from pathological changes in their skeletons is immensely useful, and offers a wealth of information on activity and workload patterns in the past (Larsen 1997). Some of the conditions considered to be associated with activity-related diseases are enthesophytes, Schmorl's nodes, DISH, and *os acromiale*.

Enthesopathies
These are characterised by ossification of ligaments and tendons producing prominent outgrowths, spurs and spicules (needles) of bone (Plate 37). Although they can be present anywhere on the skeleton, their distribution

Table 49   Percentages of observable cases with enthesophytes in both sexes

Bone	Muscle / Tendon	Male and Male?				Female and Female?			
		Right	%	Left	%	Right	%	Left	%
Radius	M. biceps	2/ 26	7.6	2/19	10.5	1/22	4.5	0/21	0
Ulna	M. triceps	8/31	25.8	7/23	30.4	2/24	8.3	1/25	4
Humerus	M.common flexor	1/29	3.4	1/24	4.1	2/25	8	0/25	0
Humerus	M.common extensor	1/29	3.4	1/24	4.1	2/26	7.6	0/26	0
Ilium	Ischial tuberosity	2/28	7.1	2/26	7.6	0/20	0	1/22	4.5
Patella	Patellar ligament	2/15	13.3	2/16	12.5	1/10	10.0	1/19	5.2
Tibia	M.quadriceps femoris	1/15	6.6	2/19	10.5	1/13	7.6	2/15	13.3
Tibia	M. soleus	1/17	5.8	1/19	5.2	0/15	0	0/17	0
Calcaneus	Achilles tendon	1/11	9.0	1/13	7.6	1/11	9.0	1/10	10

and appearance is characteristic of certain locations and they mostly show a symmetrical distribution and affect the body bilaterally (Resnick and Niwayama 1995). The skeletal analysis on the human remains from the site revealed that enthesopathies were most common in the triceps in males (*M. triceps* insertion) followed by the patella (Table 49). In the female population, the percentages were more variable because the highest numbers appeared on the right patellar ligament and on the *M. quadriceps femoris* attachment onto the left tibia (10% and 13.3%).

Schmorl's nodes
Schmorl's nodes are changes on the vertebral endplates commonly found in human remains. They represent herniations of the material of the intervertebral disc (*nucleus pulposus*) that protrude and depress the adjacent body surface (Roberts and Cox 2003). In the St Peter's population men showed a significantly higher percentage of Schmorl's nodes rather than women (p<0.05) (Table 50). This may support the hypothesis that males performed heavier and more repetitive tasks involving bending or lifting than females, which in turn led to localised trauma of the vertebral endplate.

DISH (Diffuse Idiopathic Skeletal Hyperostosis)
DISH is a skeletal disorder that generally affects males in a higher proportion than females, particularly after the age of 45 years, and is considered a type of degenerative arthritis. In the spine, the anterior longitudinal ligament ossifies (turns to bone) producing ankylosis (stiffening) in the vertebrae. This fusion does not occur in the intervertebral spaces and therefore the height between the disks is preserved (Resnick *et al* 1978) as well as the integrity of the apophyseal joints (Roberts and Manchester 1995). This pattern gives a 'flowing candle-wax appearance' to the anterior aspect of the vertebral column, particularly in the thoracic area where it is limited to the right-hand side (Rogers and Waldron

Table 50   Comparisons of the number of vertebral bodies affected in both sexes

Vertebra	M and M?	%	F and F?	%
T4	1/19	5.2	0/22	0
T5	0/17	0	2/22	9.0
T6	218	11.1	1/22	4.5
T7	8/18	44.4	2/21	9.5
T8	11/19	57.8	3/21	14.2
T9	5/17	29.4	3/21	14.2
T10	8/17	47.0	7/22	31.8
T11	7/19	36.8	6/21	28.5
T12	9/21	42.8	5/19	26.3
L1	5/22	22.7	3/21	14.2
L2	6/24	28.5	3/23	13.0
L3	3/23	13.0	1/23	4.3
L4	0/18	0	2/23	8.6
L5	0/19	0	0/21	0

1995). Although several conditions such as diabetes have been associated with its presence, social status and a rich diet seem to be the best explanatory causes for the occurrence of DISH (Waldron 1985). Only one case of DISH was identified from the site asemblage. HB 39 had vertebral fusion that took place on the right-hand side of T8–T11. This individual is also included under neoplastic conditions as he suffered from a malignant tumour.

Os acromiale
Os acromiale is a condition where the acromion (point of the shoulder) of the scapula does not fuse at the normal time (18–20 years) and therefore remains separate (Scheuer and Black 2004). It has been suggested that specific and repetitive tasks performed from a very early age might prevent the fusion from taking place (Roberts and Cox 2003). There were four cases of *os acromiale*: two middle-aged females (HB 28 and HB 88), a young male (HB 119), and a possible adult female (HB 31), which corresponds to 10.2% of the total scapulae preserved.

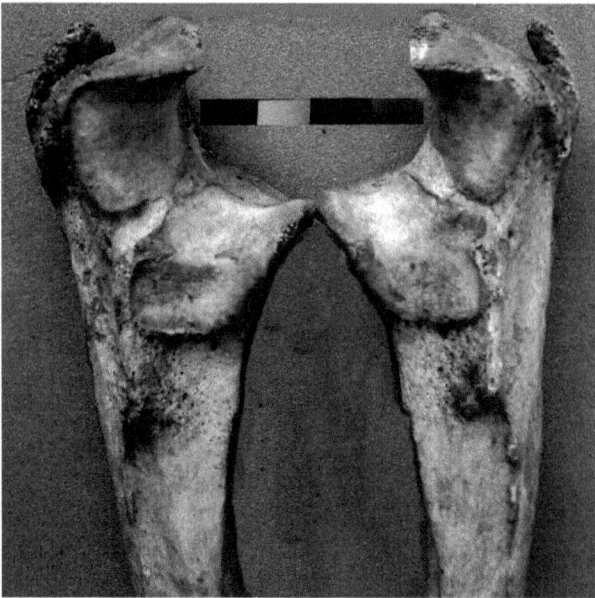

Plate 37 Triceps enthesopathies on both ulnae of HB 130

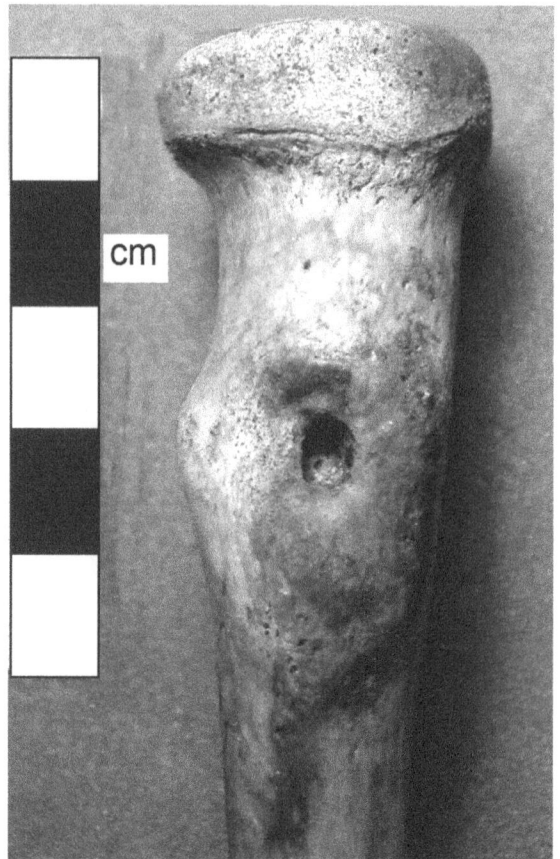

Plate 39 Cortical defect at biceps attachment on radius
of HB 119

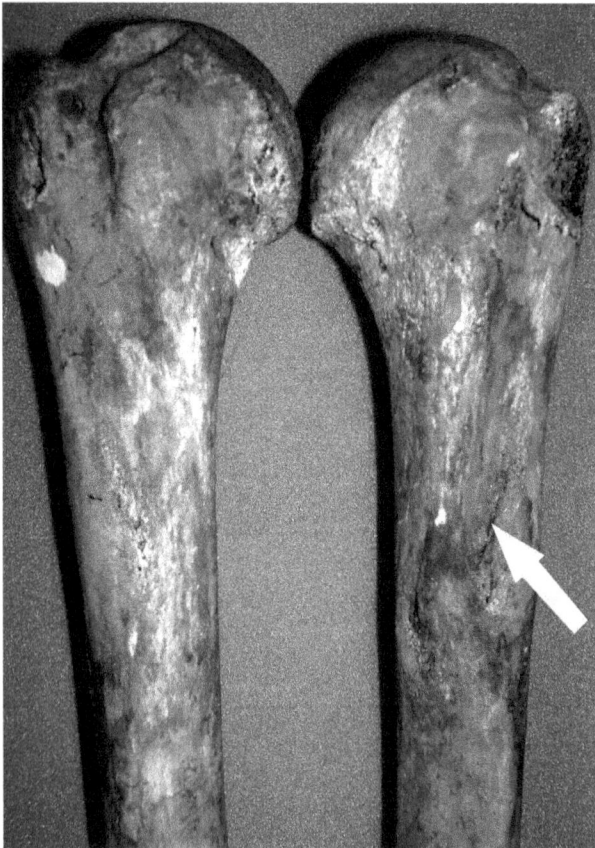

Plate 38 Cortical defect at muscle attachment (arrow)
in HB 129

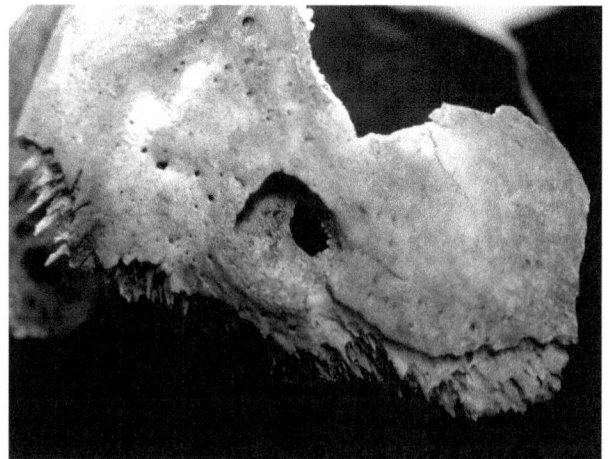

Plate 40 Cyst-like lesions on left orbit of HB 26

Miscellaneous

Three individuals from the site showed cortical defects probably as a consequence of localised trauma to the muscle. The right humerus of HB 19 and both humeri of HB 119 (Plate 38) demonstrated evidence of these types of defects. Two abnormal depressions were also found on the right radial tuberosities of HB 27 and HB 119 (Plate 39). Another miscellaneous case was HB 26 who had a perforating, cyst-like lesion with rounded margins located on the side of the left orbit just above the fronto-sphenoidal suture of unknown aetiology (Plate 40).

A COMPARISON BETWEEN ST PETER'S CHURCH, WOLVERHAMPTON, AND ST MARTIN'S CHURCH, BIRMINGHAM

A comparison of some pathologies and their crude prevalence rates (CPRs) was undertaken between the skeletal assemblage from this excavation and an assemblage of 857 burials from St Martin's, Birmingham (Brickley *et al* 2006). Both populations date to the time of the industrial revolution and they are also close to each other geographically. As a consequence of these similarities, comparison between health, status and disease may highlight similarities or differences in the lifestyles of the two groups. In order to achieve this aim, the CPR for fractures, *osteochondritis dissecans*, *cribra orbitalia*, rickets, dental pathologies, neoplasia, and joint disease were contrasted.

Fractures

The overall CPR for fractures, which includes ante mortem and perimortem fractures, from the St Peter's assemblage is 14.6%. This is less than the rate obtained for St Martin's (21.39%) but not statistically so. However, if only the adult population is considered, for St Peter's the CPR becomes 23.9%, a similar prevalence to that calculated for St Martin's cemetery. At both sites males had a higher prevalence of fractures in all age categories than females. However, the rates differ when fractures at both sites are studied by age category. At St Peter's, two age groups stand out, the young middle adult (26–35) and old middle adult (36–45), as more than a half

the individuals in these categories had at least one fracture (Table 51). By contrast, at St Martin's the number of fractures increased according to age.

From the St Peter's assemblage the highest number of fractures was evident in both sexes on the ribs, followed by the hands (Table 52). The high rate of males suffering metacarpal fractures (CPR 9.1%) is highly unusual. At St Martin's, too, as in most post-medieval sites studied, the most commonly fractured bone was the rib (2.3% of all ribs), in conjunction with the metacarpals (2.8% of the total number of metacarpals) and crush fractures of the thoracic vertebrae (2.9% of vertebrae). In populations where work was full of hazards like these, it is interesting to find a high prevalence of rib and hand fractures, since some of these lesions would be related to work accidents, in addition to crush injuries and/ or impact to the chest.

Table 51   CPR of fractures of any type by individual, sex, and age group

	No. of cases	Prevalence
Sub-adult	0/58	0 %
Adult	0/15	0 %
Adult Male	1/6	16.6 %
Adult Female	0/4	0 %
Y.A	0/0	0 %
Y. A Male	0/2	0 %
Y. A Female	0/3	0 %
Y.M.A	0/0	0 %
Y.M.A Male	3/5	60 %
Y.M.A Female	2/8	25 %
O.M.A	0/1	0 %
O.M.A Male	8/16	50 %
O.M.A Female	2/9	22.2 %
M.A	0/0	0 %
M.A Male	3/9	33.3 %
M.A Female	3/14	21.4 %
Total	22/150	14.6 %
Total (only adult individuals)	22/92	23.9 %

Other fractures like depressed fracture in the cranium or nasal fracture, both present in skeletons from St Peter's

Table 52   CPR of fractures by sex categories

Bone	Male & Male?		Female & Female?	
	No. of cases	Prevalence	No. of cases	Prevalence
Clavicle	1/37	2.7 %	0/ 39	0 %
Humerus	0/ 53	0 %	2/ 51	3.9 %
Radius	1/ 50	2 %	0/ 43	0 %
Ulna	0/ 54	0 %	1/ 49	2.04 %
Hand (metacarpals)	5/ 55	9.09 %	1/ 50	2 %
Ribs (unsided)	9/ 83	10.8 %	9/ 93	9.6 %
Femur	1/ 51	1.9 %	0/ 51	0 %
Vertebrae (unsided)	0/30	0 %	1/34	2.9 %

Table 53 CPR of osteochondritis

	No. of cases	Prevalence
Sub- adult	0/ 58	0 %
Young Adult Male	0/ 2	0 %
Young Adult Female	1/ 3	33.3 %
Young Middle Adult Male	0/ 5	0 %
Young Middle Adult Female	0/ 8	0 %
Old Middle Adult Male	2/ 16	12.5 %
Old Middle Adult Female	1/ 9	11.1 %
Old Middle Adult Unsexed	0/ 1	0 %
Mature Adult Male	0/ 9	0 %
Mature Adult Female	0/ 14	0 %
Adult Male	0/ 6	0 %
Adult Female	0/ 4	0 %
Adult Unsexed	0/ 15	0 %
Total	4/ 150	2.6 %

Table 54 CPR of individuals affected by *cribra orbitalia*

Age group	No. of affected	Prevalence	
Fetus	0	0/ 2	0 %
Neonate	0	0/ 1	0 %
Infant	0	0/ 25	0 %
Early Childhood	5	5/ 18	27.7 %
Late Childhood	1	1/ 4	25 %
Adolescent	2	2/ 8	25 %
Young Adult	0	0/ 5	0 %
Young Middle Adult	0	0/ 13	0 %
Old Middle Adult	1	1/ 26	3.8 %
Mature Adult	0	0/ 23	0 %
Adult	0	0/ 25	0 %
Total	9	9/ 150	6 %

Table 55 CPR of individuals affected by rickets

	No. of cases	Prevalence
Fetus	0/ 2	0 %
Neonate	0/ 1	0 %
Infant	1/ 25	4 %
Early Childhood	3/ 18	16.6 %
Late Childhood	0/ 4	0 %
Adolescent	0/ 8	0 %
Young Adult	0/ 5	0 %
Young Middle Adult	0/ 13	0 %
Old Middle Adult	0/ 26	0 %
Mature Adult	1/ 23	4.3 %
Adult	0/ 25	0 %
Total	5/ 150	3.3 %

and St Martin's, are more likely to be associated with interpersonal violence (Roberts and Cox 2003).

Osteochondritis dissecans

Osteochondritis dissecans, like fracture, is indicative of a traumatic event. Comparing the CPR from the two post-medieval sites, a similar rate is found, 2.6% at St Peter's and 2.7% at St Martin's. However, differences start to appear when the prevalence is studied by sex category. In the St Martin's assemblage, males were more frequently affected than females. From St Peter's, prevalence is the same for males and females (Table 53). When the location of the condition on the skeleton is studied, more differences become evident. Although the most commonly involved location was the elbow joint at both sites, at St Martin's a significant difference between sides was recorded, with the right side more frequently affected than the left. By contrast, at St Peter's there were no side differences, since both were affected to a similar extent.

Cribra orbitalia

From the St Peter's assemblage, *cribra orbitalia* was found in eight sub-adults, representing 13.7% of the entire juvenile group. Only one case was recorded in the adult population, a 36–45-year-old male. Consequently the CPR for the entire population is 6%, a lower rate than the 9.64% obtained for St Martin's (Table 54) but not statistically so. Even the adult cases with *cribra orbitalia* had a higher prevalence at the latter site.

According to the study conducted by Roberts and Cox (2003), the CPR for *cribra orbitalia* at other post-medieval sites is very variable, the highest being found at Newcastle Infirmary (24.87%) while the lowest was seen at Kingston-upon-Thames (0.28%). As a result, the rates found on the two sites were in the expected range. By contrast, the CPR of 34% of those whose crania survived at Spitalfields seems unusually high.

According to Cox (1998), the iron deficiency itself is related to anaemic mothers, especially those who bore several children in quick succession. This would explain the higher rate of females manifesting *cribra orbitalia* compared to males at St Martin's, notably the young adults. In addition, *cribra orbitalia* may also be associated with infant feeding practices such as giving 'pap' or 'panada' (a mixture of water and flour) which was substituted for breast milk. This practice, certainly, did not help to nourish the infants adequately, which would lead to a poorer immune system, as well as a higher risk of contracting intestinal parasites such as worms (Roberts and Cox 2003).

Rickets

According to the study carried out by Roberts and Cox (2003), the mean CPR for rickets at Victorian sites is 3.65%, a prevalence similar to the 3.3% found in the St Peter's assemblage (Table 55). By contrast, the CPR for St Martin's is higher, with 7.5% of the entire population affected. However, this higher prevalence is probably due to the additional techniques used to diagnose the presence of the disease.

Table 56   Number of individuals affected by dental pathologies (permanent dentition)

Pathologies	Caries		Abscess*		Calculus		DEH		Periodontal disease	
	No. of cases	CPR	No. of cases	CPR	No. of cases	CPR	No. of cases	CPR	No. of cases	CPR
Sub-adult	3/ 8	37.5	0/ 8	0	3/ 8	37.5	3/ 8	37.5	0/ 8	0
Adult	0/ 2	0	0/ 2	0	0/ 2	0	0/ 2	0	0/ 2	0
Adult Male	2/ 2	100	0/ 2	0	2/ 2	100	1/ 2	50	2/ 2	100
Adult Female	1/ 2	50	0/ 2	0	1/ 2	50	1/ 2	50	0/ 2	0
Y.A	0/ 0	0	0/ 0	0	0/ 0	0	0/ 0	0	0/ 0	0
Y. A Male	1/ 2	50	0/ 2	0	1/ 2	50	2/ 2	100	0/ 2	0
Y. A Female	0/ 1	0	0/ 1	0	1/ 1	100	1/ 1	100	0/ 1	0
Y.M.A	0/ 0	0	0/ 0	0	0/ 0	0	0/ 0	0	0/ 0	0
Y.M.A Male	4/ 5	80	1/ 5	20	4/ 5	80	5/ 5	100	1/ 5	20
Y.M.A Female	5/ 6	83.3	2/ 6	33.3	4/ 6	66.6	5/ 6	83.3	2/ 6	33.3
O.M.A	0/ 0	0	0/ 0	0	0/ 0	0	0/ 0	0	0/ 0	0
O.M.A Male	9/ 11	81.8	6/ 11	54.5	9/ 11	81.8	9/ 11	81.8	5/ 11	45.4
O.M.A Female	5/ 7	71.4	1/ 7	14.2	3/ 7	42.8	3/ 7	42.8	0/ 7	0
M.A	0/ 0	0	0/ 0	0	0/ 0	0	0/ 0	0	0/ 0	0
M.A Male	6/ 8	75	6/ 8	75	6/ 8	75	5/ 8	62.5	4/ 8	50
M.A Female	9/ 11	81.8	1/ 11	9.09	9/ 11	81.8	3/ 11	27.2	4/ 11	36.3
Total	45/65	69.2	17/65	26.1	43/65	66.1	38/65	58.4	18/65	27.6

*Granulomas are included within the abscess

The highest prevalence of rickets at the two sites is concentrated in the children from 0 to three years of age. Vitamin D deficiency was a common condition in the 19th century, especially in industrial and mining areas (Lewis 1999). Cities were over-populated, with streets that were narrow, polluted and full of smoke due to a rapid increase in industrialisation. This prevented sunlight from reaching the children's skin and produced an increase in cases of rickets. Infant feeding practices, as well as the quality and quantity of dairy products available at the market, also made young children prone to develop vitamin D deficiency.

Dental pathologies

An analysis of the CPR for caries, abscesses, calculus, dental enamel hypoplasia and periodontal disease was carried out for all of the individuals with preserved dentitions (Table 56).

Caries

Looking at the prevalence rates for caries in the two groups it is evident that caries is higher in the skeletons from St Peter's, with 69.2% of individuals affected, compared to 51.3% at St Martin's (p<0.0773). The number of those with caries increases according to age category at both sites, although sometimes older individuals can have a slightly lower prevalence than the previous age category. However, these lower levels may be related to ante mortem tooth loss. Furthermore, of the two groups, females are more likely to be affected, although the difference is not statistically significant. The first molar is the most frequently affected tooth at both sites. The high increase in the incidence of caries during the 19th century is associated with the elevated consumption of refined flours, fermentable carbohydrates and sugar (Mays 1998). This is corroborated by the results from the two cemeteries. As a consequence it is possible to deduce that the intake and accessibility of these products was similar in both places.

Abscesses

The number of tooth sockets (TPR) affected by abscesses at St Peter's (2.1%) is similar to that at St Martin's (2.63%). The figure from St Peter's is even closer when

Table 57   CPR of abscesses by number of teeth affected

	Male & Male?		Female & Female?		Adult*		Sub-adult deciduous		Total	
	n	%	n	%	n	%	n	%	n	%
Total teeth	527	69.3	383	60.5	234	98.7	408	85.7	1552	100
Abscesses	23	4.3	10	1.8	0	0	0	0	33	2.1

only the adults are studied, 2.8% (Table 57). Most of the abscesses were located in the upper jaw, in both cases, since the maxilla is less robust than the mandible and consequently more prone to develop these perforations. From the St Peter's assemblage there is a marked difference between the sexes (4.3% for the males, as opposed to 1.8% for females). This is not the case at St Martin's, where there is no particular difference between the sexes.

Calculus

There are a lot of similarities between the two sites when the total number of individuals with calculus (CPR) is analysed, although the prevalence is significantly higher (p<0.001) at St Martin's (76.8%) than at St Peter's (66.1%). As with many other dental pathologies, calculus increases with age. The results at both sites support this observation. Looking at differences between the sexes, it is clear that males show a higher prevalence of calculus than females. At St Martin's a difference was also found between those buried in earth-cut graves and those disposed of in vaults. The individuals from the earth-cut graves showed a higher prevalence than the other group. However, whether this difference between occupants of the two types of grave at St Martin's is due to diet or oral hygiene is not clear.

Dental Enamel Hypoplasia (DEH)

DEH is the only dental pathology that decreases in prevalence with age, as corroborated by the results at the two sites. The number of individuals affected, 58.4%, is smaller at St Peter's than the 69% found at St Martin's. While at St Martin's women are more affected than men, at St Peter's the males are more likely to be involved. The canine is the most frequently affected tooth by far at both sites. Since this tooth develops between six months and seven years of age, it could be suggested that this was the most common time to suffer an episode of severe malnutrition or high fever.

Periodontal disease

There is a strong correlation between age and an increase in periodontal disease at both sites. The CPR at St Martin's, with 50% of the entire population showing signs of periodontal disease, is nearly double that seen at St Peter's (27.6%). This difference is related to the fact that a different method was used in the recording of the disease for the population at St Peter's. The scoring system for different degrees of severity was based on Ogden's (unpublished) methodology. In this technique the alveolar margin is observed and the length of the root is irrelevant, since this is related to compensatory eruption.

The pattern of caries and calculus demonstrates similarities between the two cemeteries, although St Martin's shows differences between the earth-cut and vault burials. It is clear from these results that access to refined food and sugar was a factor at both sites, in addition to problems related to dental hygiene. Moreover, females had better dental hygiene at both sites.

Table 58 CPR of neoplasia

	No. of cases	Prevalence
Sub- adult	0/ 58	0 %
Young Adult Male	0/ 2	0 %
Young Adult Female	0/ 3	0 %
Young Middle Adult Male	0/ 5	0 %
Young Middle Adult Female	0/ 8	0 %
Old Middle Adult Male	3/ 16	18.75 %
Old Middle Adult Female	0/ 9	0 %
Old Middle Adult Unsexed	0/ 1	0 %
Mature Adult Male	3/ 9	33.3 %
Mature Adult Female	1/ 14	7.1 %
Adult Male	0/ 6	0 %
Adult Female	0/ 4	0 %
Adult Unsexed	0/ 15	0 %
Total	7/ 150	4.6 %

Neoplasia

The CPR for St Martin's of 3.23% for all cases of neoplasia is less than the 4.6% obtained for St Peter's (Table 58). Nevertheless these rates are high if they are compared with the mean prevalence of 0.30% for Victorian sites calculated by Roberts and Cox (2003). This finding is very significant for the study of cancer in past populations. The high prevalence at the two sites may be related to two factors: firstly, the excellent preservation of the skeletons, especially in the St Peter's assemblage, where it was possible to record 'sunburst lesions' on the spine of one individual. However, osteosarcoma of the spine is a very unusual finding, even in modern populations. Second, it may be related to the presence of a considerable number of mature adults who lived long enough to develop and manifest the disease on their bones, since neoplastic disease is found mainly in old people. It is also likely that the environmental (atmospheric pollution) and living/ working conditions of these two groups would have made them susceptible to develop this condition.

Joint disease

The number of individuals affected by osteoarthritis of the spine at St Peter's (31.25%) is high compared to the CPR at St Martin's (19.59%), probably due to the small size of the sample at the former site and a larger proportion having attained an advanced age at the former site. The location of the lesions is also different. Whereas at St Martin's the most frequently affected vertebral region are T3–T5 and L3–L5, at St Peter's the cervical region, especially C1–C2, and C4, shows more osteoarthritic vertebrae (Table 59).

However, when osteoarthritis of other joints is compared, the CPR at St Martin's (21.7% for females and 24.6% for

Table 59   CPR of spinal OA in males and females (all the vertebrae affected and all the vertebrae present)

Vertebrae	No. of cases (Males)	Prevalence (Males)	No. of cases (Females)	Prevalence	No. of cases (Total)	Prevalence (Total)
C1	5/24	20.8 %	1/25	4 %	6/49	12.2 %
C2	4/25	16 %	3/21	14.2 %	7/46	15.2 %
C3	2/22	9.09 %	2/21	9.5 %	4/43	9.3 %
C4	2/22	9.09 %	3/23	13.04 %	5/45	11.1 %
C5	0/22	0 %	3/21	14.2 %	3/43	6.9 %
C6	0/21	0 %	0/22	0 %	0/43	0 %
C7	1/22	4.5 %	0/19	0 %	1/41	2.4 %
T1	2/21	9.5 %	0/20	0 %	2/41	4.8 %
T2	0/19	0 %	1/22	4.5 %	1/41	2.4 %
T3	1/19	5.2 %	1/22	4.5 %	2/41	4.8 %
T4	2/19	10.5 %	2/22	9.09 %	4/41	9.7 %
T5	1/17	5.8 %	2/22	9.09 %	3/39	7.6 %
T6	3/18	16.6 %	0/22	0 %	3/40	7.5 %
T7	1/18	5.5 %	0/21	0 %	1/39	2.5 %
T8	2/19	10.5 %	0/21	0 %	2/40	5 %
T9	1/17	5.8 %	1/21	4.7 %	2/38	5.2 %
T10	2/17	11.7 %	2/22	9.09 %	4/39	10.2 %
T11	1/19	5.2 %	1/21	4.7 %	2/40	5 %
T12	0/21	0 %	2/19	10.5 %	2/40	5 %
L1	0/22	0 %	0/21	0 %	0/43	0 %
L2	0/21	0 %	1/23	4.3 %	1/44	2.2 %
L3	0/23	0 %	2/23	8.6 %	2/46	4.3 %
L4	1/18	5.5 %	2/23	8.6 %	3/41	7.3 %
L5	1/19	5.2 %	2/21	9.5 %	3/40	7.5 %

Table 60   CPR of non-spinal OA in males, females, and unsexed of different age groups

	Male		Female		Unsexed		Total	
	No. of cases	%	No. of cases	%	No. of cases	%	No. of cases	%
Young Adult	0/ 2	0	0/ 3	0	0/ 0	0	0/ 5	0
Young Middle Adult	0/ 5	0	3/ 8	37.5	0/ 0	0	3/ 13	23.07
Old Middle Adult	3/ 16	18.75	2/ 9	22.2	0/ 1	0	5/ 26	19.2
Mature Adult	5/ 9	55.5	2/ 14	14.2	0/ 0	0	7/ 23	30.4
Adult	2/ 6	33.3	1/ 4	25	0/ 15	0	3/ 25	12
Total	10/ 38	26.3	8/ 38	21.05	0/ 16	0	18/ 92	19.5

Table 61   CPR of individuals affected by non-spinal OA according to the joint affected

Joint	Male and Male?				Female and Female?			
	Right	%	Left	%	Right	%	Left	%
Temporo-mandibular	1/26	4	0/26	0	0/27	0	0/27	0
Gleno-humeral	2/22	9	2/25	8	0/22	0	1/23	4.3
Acromio-clavicular	4/17	23.5	3/20	15	0/19	0	1/16	6.2
Elbow	1/29	3.4	1/24	4.1	2/25	8	1/26	3.8
Hand*	5/30	16.6	4/25	16	4/25	16	4/25	16
Costo-clavicular	0/27	0	1/27	3.7	0/27	0	0/27	0
Costo-manubrial	0/27	0	0/27	0	0/27	0	1/27	3.7
Costo-vertebral	0/27	0	0/27	0	4/27	14.8	0/27	0
Hip	0/28	0	1/21	4.7	0/20	0	0/22	0
Knee	0/23	0	0/21	0	1/17	5.8	0/21	0
Foot*	4/14	29	1/14	7.1	2/14	14.2	0/12	0

*one or more joints

females) is similar to that at St Peter's (26% for males and 21% for females), although the frequencies are almost reversed between the sexes (Table 60). One of the conditions that increases the risk of developing OA is age. As the age of the individual increases, the chances of OA are higher. This is obvious in the individuals affected by OA from St Martin's. However, at St Peter's the frequency of OA does not increase steadily with age. In this sample the prevalence recorded in young middle adult individuals is higher than the old middle adult one. Therefore another cause must be sought for the development of OA in this age group. Although there are plenty of factors which influence this condition, such as sex, metabolism, nutrition of the articular cartilage, hormones or heredity, physical activity and mechanical stress seems a more reasonable explanation in this case.

There is no particular difference between the sexes, although at St Martin's females showed a greater frequency of OA. The most commonly affected skeletal regions at both sites were the clavicle and the joints of the hands. In contrast, at St Martin's the knee (distal femur) also showed a high frequency, whereas at St Peter's the foot joints were badly affected (Table 61). This suggests that there may be different factors influencing the rates of OA at the two sites. Whereas the St Peter's population have some cases caused by mechanical stress or physical activity, the individuals affected by OA at St Martin's are related to age. At Spitalfields osteoarthritis is also correlated with age and the joints most likely to be affected are the shoulder (including the acromioclavicular joint), the hand and the spine. This situation is very similar to that found in the assemblage from St Peter's.

CHAPTER 6

The Families

Sarah Watt

During the excavations, six legible or partly legible grave memorials and four legible or partly legible *depositum* plates were discovered. In each case the information was incomplete but since the church records do not specify the exact location of the burials, ie whether they were in the churchyard or the burial ground, this was the only source of information that positively identified some people interred in the burial ground. It was important therefore to find out as much as possible about these named individuals, and their families, and in doing so place them in context in 19th-century Wolverhampton.

Of the *depositum* plates recovered from burials only two had sufficient information for further research.

There were some fragments of grave memorials found in five of the seven vaults. However, only some yielded significant information. The grave memorials in the vaults may or may not have been associated with the human bones in the vaults, as it is possible that they were used as backfill during the 1970's clearance operation. However, given the later dates associated with the Carter and Fullwood families, it is highly likely that they were buried in a vault since burials in the open graveyard appears to have ceased around 1850.

Two further grave memorials were recovered during the excavation through the burial ground soil. Although they were unstratified, the memorials showing the names Vale and Mansell were investigated.

Figure 13 illustrates the locations of some of the key streets mentioned in this chapter.

DEPOSITUM PLATES

James Whit...
The following inscription was recorded on a *depositum* plate for HB 70:

'James Whit...
Died May 20th 1827
Aged 42'

The burial records indicate that this individual was James White, who was buried on May 24th 1827. According to an 1818–20 directory, he was a grocer and tea dealer operating from Dudley Street. Mr White had evidently had a stressful childhood. His teeth displayed one of the severest cases of dental enamel hypoplasma (a defect in the development of tooth enamel during childhood resulting from malnutrition or stress) and his limb bones showed clear evidence of rickets (vitamin D deficiency) (see Chapter 5).

William Brise
A partial inscription on a *depositum* plate associated with HB 36 records this man's death on 22/1/18. An examination of the IGI and NBI did not reveal any further information.

Rachel
This plate was associated with HB 20. The lack of information prevented further research.

...aylis
This plate was associated with HB 140. The surname was incomplete but could relate to Baylis. However no further research was possible.

GRAVE MEMORIALS

Unstratified
The Mansell Family
This grave memorial was found unstratified in the burial ground soil. Only a partial inscription could be deciphered, that being the surname Mansell, and the second part of a fore or middle name, reading (possibly) '-ariah'. The date of death (4/?/1832) meant that it could perhaps refer to a Samuel Mansell, who is shown on the burial records for St Peter's to have been buried on 8/4/1832. This could perhaps be the case if he had a second name compatible with the partial information on the memorial, for instance 'Zachariah'. Samuel Mansell died at the age of 44. In 1792, another Samuel Mansell, perhaps a relation, is listed in the Rates as a huckster (purveyor of provisions) at 7 Bell Street. In 1805 and 1818 there was a Samuel Mansell, rule maker, at 19 Salop Street, who may have been the individual referred to on the memorial. No further information was found, as these dates are pre-census.
The Vale Family
The following inscription came from a grave memorial found unstratified in the burial ground soil;

'Sacred
To? the memory of
Margaret Wife of Charles Vale
Who departed this life March 29th 1824

Charles...'

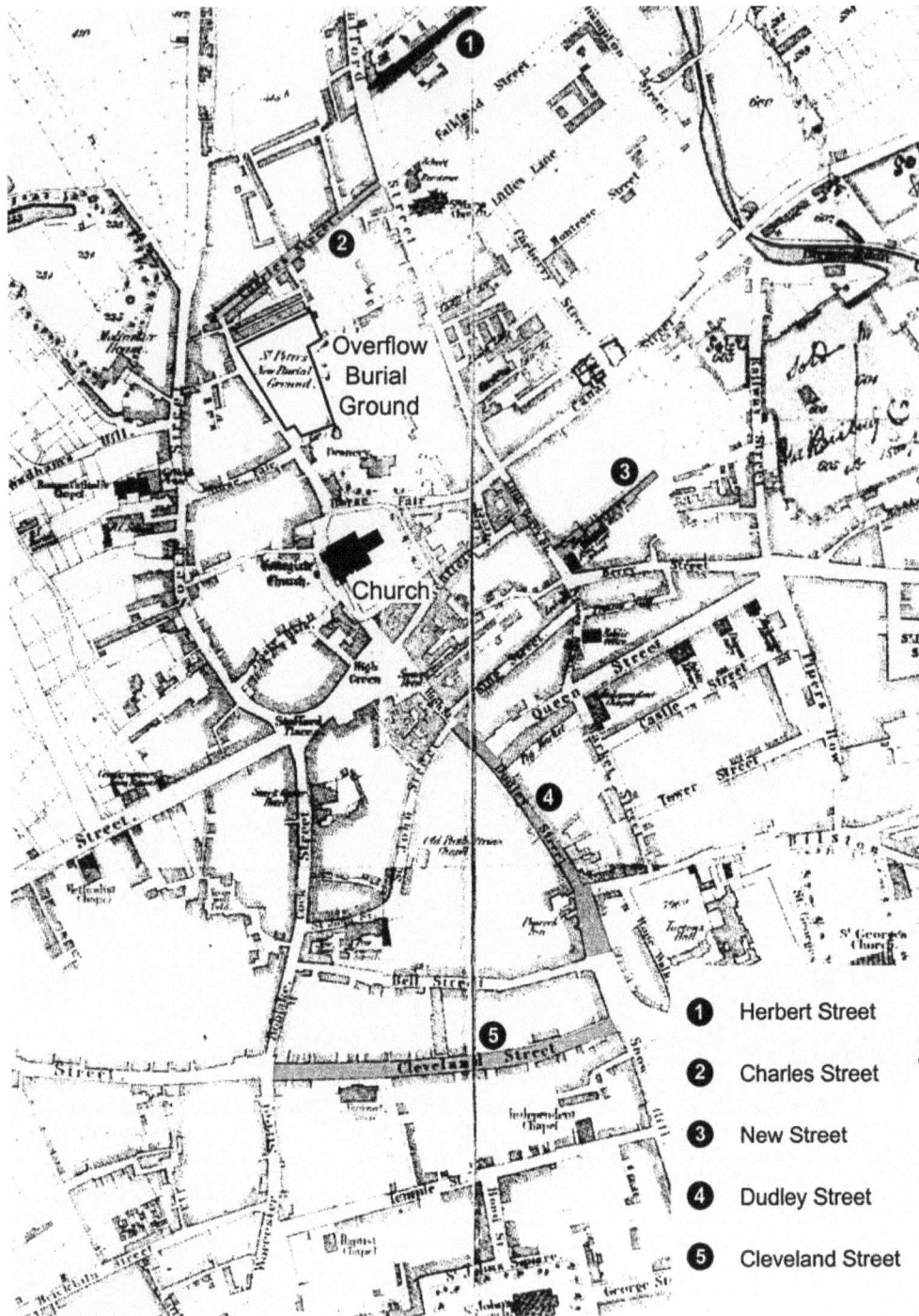

Figure 13 Map showing the location of key streets mentioned in Chapter 6

Charles and Margaret Vale were both identified on one grave memorial. Margaret died at the age of 61 in 1824, and was buried on 1/4/1824. Charles Vale died seven years later on the 10th September 1831. Trade directories from 1805 and 1818 list a Charles Vale, brass case lock (or rim lock) manufacturer, at No. 4 New Street.

Vault 1
One fragment of grave memorial was found that had the name 'Collins' inscribed on it. No further research was possible.

Vault 2
Two fragments of grave memorial were found here with only partial legible inscriptions. On one it was only possible to read 'September' and the age (74) so no further research was possible. On the other, the partial name 'J. Bag... who died in 18..', was visible. Examination of the burial records revealed that this could be J Baggerley, Baggott, Bagley or Bagnall.

Vault 3
No grave memorials with discernible names were found.

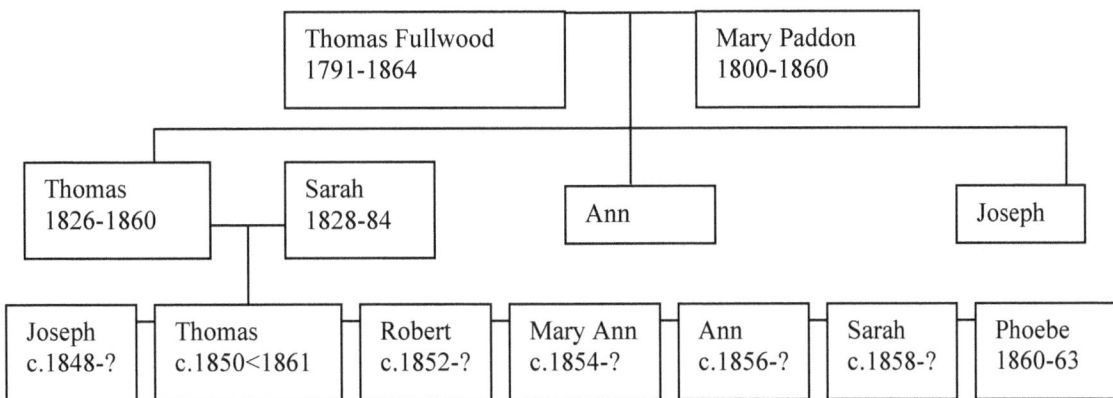

Figure 14 The Fullwood Family tree

Vault 4

There were five fragments of grave memorial found one of which was inscribed 'T Ford'. An examination of the IGI and NBI did not provide any further information, so no other information research was possible.

Vault 5

The Fullwood Family

A grave memorial to three members of this family was found in Vault 5 but was not associated with particular burials. It read:

'In memory of
Thomas Fullwood
died October 25th 1864
aged 73 years
Mary wife of the above
died July 5th 1860,
aged 60 years
Thomas Fullwood
Son of the above died March 19th 1860
aged 34 years
Prepare to meet thy God'

There was also a fragment of another stone in the vault, bearing the name Samuel, although no Samuel Fullwood was encountered during the research for this report. This may indicate that this stone, and possibly the Fullwood stone, did not originally come from this vault. However, it is also possible that the partial remains of the separate burials (HB 12a, 12b, 13a, 13b,and 14) could be the remains of members of the Fullwood family. They are all children, infants and young adults.

An examination of the birth, marriage and burial records of St Peter's reveal that there were several branches of the Fullwood or Fulwood family living in the town in the late 18th and 19th century. Entries in all the registers indicate a close association with the church.

First generation – Thomas and Mary (Fig 14)
The IGI lists the marriage of Thomas Fullwood and Mary Paddon at St Peter's on 6th December 1817, and nine

children are recorded in the birth register, with three being baptised at one time, possibly to save money. Large families were not uncommon at this time, but the Fullwood family was also an illustration of the high infant mortality rate, with at least three children dying before they reached their fifth birthday. In 1851 Thomas Fullwood was working as a screw maker, employing six men. At this time, only Joseph, their youngest child, was still living in the family home, along with a brother-in-law, who worked as a locksmith, and a 16-year-old apprentice locksmith from Penkridge. At the time of the 1861 census, Thomas Fullwood Senior lived at 30 Charles Street and was working as a whitesmith, despite being 70 years old. A whitesmith was a tin-plate worker. Joseph, aged 23, was still unmarried and living at home. Mary died on 5th July 1860 at the age of 60, and was buried four days later in the 'overflow' burial ground for St Peter's Church. Thomas died four years later on the 25th October, at the age of 73. At the time of his death he lived at Herbert Street, probably with his widowed daughter and family, since his granddaughter Phoebe was also living there when she died aged three the year before. Subsequently, his daughter-in-law Sarah must have moved because she is listed as living in Lord Street when she died in 1884.

Second generation – Thomas (junior), Ann and Joseph
The eldest child, Thomas, had left home by 1851, when he would have been 25 years old. He also worked as a whitesmith. He married Sarah, with whom he had seven children, Joseph, Thomas, Robert, Mary Ann, Ann, Sarah and Phoebe. However, Sarah was widowed in March, 1860; her husband died prematurely on the 25th October at the age of 34, leaving her to look after six children aged 13, nine, seven, five, three and one respectively. Thomas must have died shortly after the birth of Phoebe, and the burial records for the parish of St Peter's state that he was 'of Charles Street'. The 1861 census shows their address to be Court No. 3, Charles Street. Thomas died of 'apoplexy', after six hours, as stated on the death certificate (Fig 15). Joseph Fullwood, either his brother or his son, was present at the death. The Oxford English Dictionary lists apoplexy as 'a malady, very sudden in its

HC 820991

**CERTIFIED COPY of an
Pursuant to the Births and**

**ENTRY OF DEATH
Deaths Registration Act 1953**

	Registration District Wolverhampton								
1860 .	**Death in the Sub-district of**	Wolverhampton East				in the County of Stafford			
Columns: -	1	2	3	4	5	6	7	8	9
No.	When and where died	Name and surname	Sex	Age	Occupation	Cause of death	Signature, description, and residence of informant	When registered	Signature of registrar
208	Nineteenth March 1860 Charles Street	Thomas FULLWOOD	Male	34 years	Whitesmith and son of Thomas FULLWOOD a Whitesmith	Apoplexy 6 hours Certified	Joseph Fullwood Present at the death Charles Street Wolverhampton	Twentieth March 1869	F P Fellows Registrar.

Certified to be a true copy of an entry in a register in my custody.

_____ _annudun_ _____ _Superintendent Registrar_

7th June 2002 _Date_

Figure 15 Copy of death certificate for Thomas Fullwood 1860

attack, which arrests more or less completely the powers of sense and motion; it is usually caused by an effusion of blood or serum in the brain, and preceded by giddiness, partial loss of muscular power, etc'. It is impossible to say what caused such a sudden illness. This seems to be equivalent, in modern terms, to a stroke.

Thomas and Sarah's second son, Thomas, who was one year old in 1851, does not appear on the 1861 census, so he may have died in infancy. It would appear that the premature death of the children's father led to his eldest son, Joseph, having to work as a whitesmith by the age of 13, following the family trade. The trade directory for 1851 lists two Thomas Fullwoods on Charles Street, a tin-plate worker and a wood-screw maker. Thomas Fullwood, the wood-screw manufacturer, was operating from 22 Temple Street in 1818, and is listed at Charles Street in 1834 and, again, as a stove-screw maker at Charles Street in 1845.

Vault 6
The Carter Family
The following inscription came from a grave memorial in Vault 6, but was not associated with a burial:

'Sacred to the memory
of

John Carter
Who departed this life April 10th 1864
aged 56 years
Also of
Mary Carter
Relict of the above
Who died April 3rd 1877
Aged 60 years
Also of
Thomas Watwood Carter
Son of the above
Who died November 1st 1871
Aged 15 years
Therefore be ye also ready for in such an
Hour as ye think not the son of man comes'

First generation (Fig 16)
As it is clear from the various documents consulted that two families with the name Carter lived on Charles Street in Wolverhampton (Plate 41) between 1841 and 1861, it is probably reasonable to surmise that they comprised two generations of the same family. The John Carter of the second generation is the man recorded on the grave memorial, but it is likely that the people described in this first section are his parents, as their respective ages would allow this to be the case. The John Carter of the first generation was about 55 at the time of the 1841 census, at

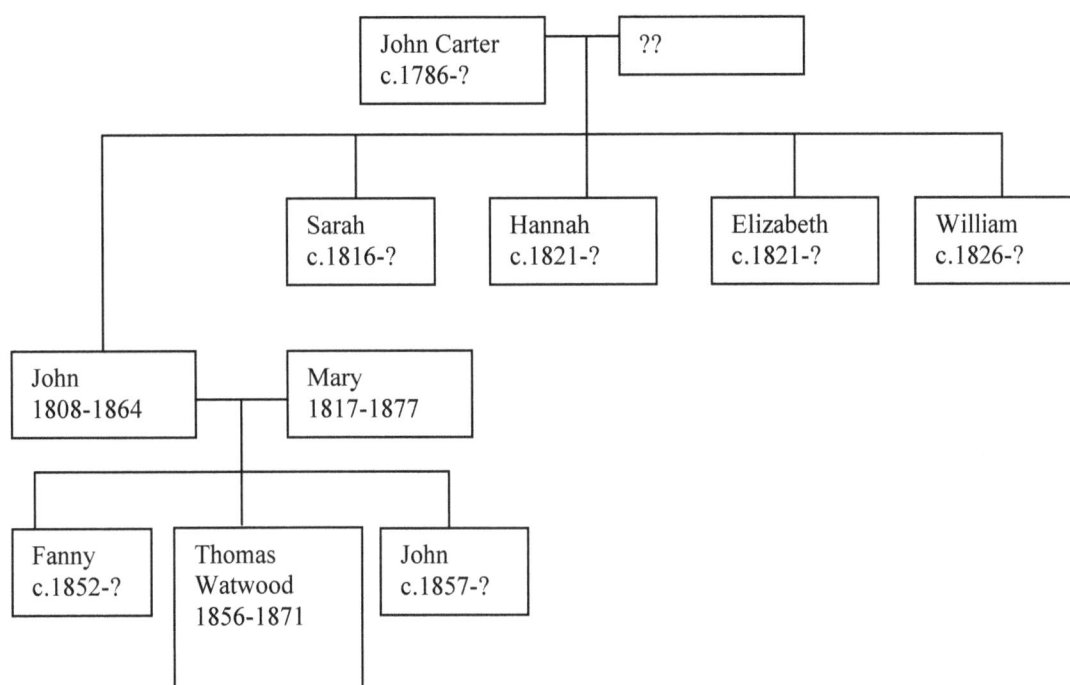

Figure 16 Partial family tree for John Carter

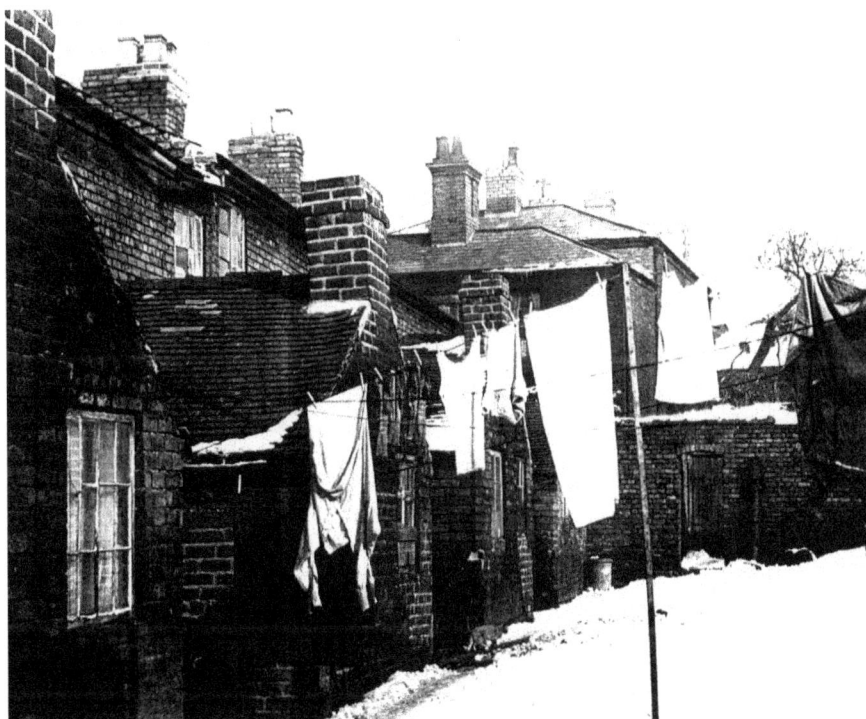

Plate 41 Charles Street 1841–1861

which time he was working as a tin-plate worker. It appears that he had been widowed by this time, although this is not explicitly stated, and was living with his daughter, Sarah, 25, a 'seampstress', Hannah, 20, also a 'seampstress', Elizabeth, ?20, and William, 15. It is not clear but it is probable that Hannah, Elizabeth and William were also his children. By 1851, when John Carter's age was given (inexplicably) as 69, and he is stated to be a widower, he was living only with his daughter Sarah, who remained unmarried. It is not known when John died. If the John Carter described in the following section was indeed his son, he would not have appeared on the census because he would have been 33 in 1841 and had presumably already left home.

Second generation

The John Carter of the grave memorial was born around 1808 and died in 1864. He married Mary, who was born

75

around 1817 and died in 1877. They may have married relatively late, as they do not appear to have had children until the 1850s, when they had Fanny (1852), Thomas Watwood (1856) and John Thomas (1857). In 1861, John Carter was working as a beerhouse keeper, and the family lived at No. 49 Charles Street. However, his son Thomas Watwood is not listed on the census for this year. Thomas Watwood in fact died at the age of 15 in 1871, so should still be listed on the census. Also living with the family in 1861 was Fanny Morris, a 15-year-old unmarried servant from Leicester.

A John Carter, beer retailer, is listed on Charles Street in trade directories from 1845 and 1851. There is also a reference in a collection held at Wolverhampton Archives to Mary Carter, a victualler, in 1868. In an 1869 directory she is listed under Inns and Taverns at 'The Broom Girl'. She had presumably taken over her husband's occupation after his death in 1864. There are several more references to her in regard to mortgages and conveyances of property in Wolverhampton in Graiseley Row, Brickkiln Street, North Road, Bennetts Fold, Derry Street, Oxford Street, Mill Street and Canal Street, where she appeared to have a share in various houses and messuages. A related reference is made to an Inland Revenue legacy receipt on the estate of Mary Carter late of Dudley, Worcestershire, 4th October 1877; it is known that Mary died the day before this date. Her third child John is also referred to as 'John Thomas Carter of Wolverhampton, grocer's assistant, who had a fifth share in some property including a dwellinghouse in Bennetts Fold in December 1877'.

John Carter's probate will, dated 9th September 1863, is held in Wolverhampton Archives. This was dated exactly seven months before his death, and it is clear from his death certificate that he had been ill for a year beforehand. The cause of death is recorded as 'phthisis'. This appears to have been a term used for pulmonary consumption, 'a disease of the lungs…characterised by progressive consolidation of the pulmonary texture, and by the subsequent softening and disintegration of the consolidated tissue' (OED). A contemporary quotation (Allbutt 1898) states that 'in several towns the phthisis death rate had undergone a notable decrease since the introduction of an improved system of sewerage'. Varieties of the disease were common amongst colliers, grinders and even potters, it being brought on by the deposition of various industrial dusts and particles in the lungs. Presumably, it could also have been caused by damp conditions and the general industrial air pollution created by the mass production of coal and iron in the area, given that John Carter worked as a beer retailer. Of course, it is also possible that he had been involved in such industries when he was younger.

He had appointed his wife Mary and her brother Joseph Harriman, an iron brazier, as joint executors of his estate (interestingly, two Harriman households, the heads of which were both iron braziers, lived on Charles Street at

Nos 47 and 49 in 1861, although a Joseph is not listed, as he may have left the family home by this date). He left several messuages and dwellinghouses in North Road, Oxley Street, Brickkiln Street, and Graiseley Row, from which rents and profits were to be received by Harriman and paid to Mary for the support of herself and their children and, after her death, to be held in trust for his 'three children, Fanny Carter, John Thomas Carter and Thomas Watwood Carter'. His personal estate and effects, including stock in trade furniture and utensils, were also to go to Harriman 'to permit and suffer my wife to receive the profits of the same'. He also stated 'my son Thomas Watwood Carter if he lives to attain the age of fourteen years a sum of £50 will become payable under a policy of assurance for his benefit', also directing that 'my trustee and executor and also my executor…do receive the same if it shall become payable as aforesaid and lay such sum out at interest until my son Thomas Watwood Carter shall attain his age of twenty-one years and then pay the principal of such sum and interest that may accrue from the same unto him for his own use'. Sadly, Thomas Watwood Carter died at the age of 15, on the 1st November 1871, after suffering from diarrhoea for 14 days, so would never have received his inheritance.

He and his wife appear to have owned shares in property on various streets in the town, although some of these were in the slum areas. Plate 42 shows an area gripped by poverty and poor housing, which may well have been the same housing in use 100 years before.

This information from his will, together with the fact that he employed a servant, would suggest that he was comparatively well off. In addition, if the vault in which his grave memorial was discovered was purchased for the use of his family, this would also suggest a degree of wealth and status in the community.

Trades and Occupations

John Carter's occupation as a beer retailer is not entirely clear. He is not listed in trade directories under Inns and Taverns, but under Beerhouses in 1858 and under Beer Retailers in 1860. His death certificate gives his occupation as a Retail Brewer, and he died in the 'Buy a Broom Inn' on Charles Street, presumably his place of abode. Curiously, this inn is not listed in any of the Trade Directories consulted. The aforementioned 'Broom Girl' listed under Mary Carter in 1869 may have been the same inn with a slight change of name, but no prior reference was found for this either. A beer retailer may have operated from a shop, as the equivalent of today's off-licences, rather than from an inn. Although the death certificate lists him as a Retail Brewer, he does not appear to have been in the trade directories under 'Brewers'. Mary Carter worked as a victualler, presumably carrying on her husband's occupation as a beerhouse keeper after his death. A victualler was someone who provided food and drink for payment, and can refer to the keeper of an eating-house or inn.

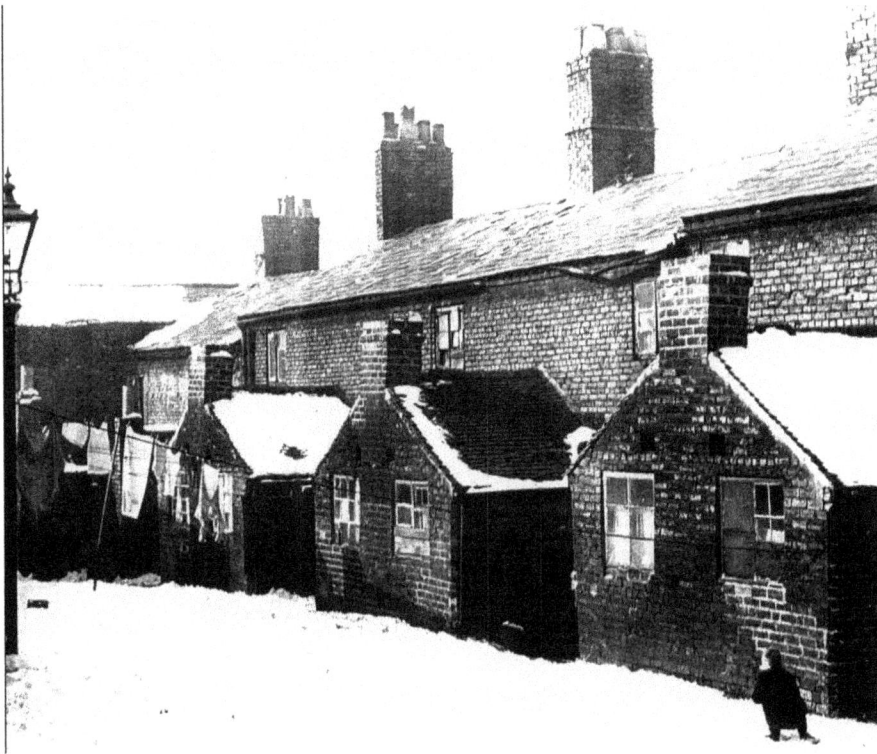

Plate 42 Charles Street 1950s

The other individuals mentioned above had various trades and occupations common in 19th-century Wolverhampton.

Samuel Mansell worked as a huckster in 1792. A huckster was a retailer of small goods, either in a small shop or on a stall. The term also covers pedlars and hawkers (and could also be used as a term of reproach in reference to someone who made profit in a mean or petty way, or who acted as a broker or middleman).

Whitesmithing, a trade practised by both Thomas Fullwoods, the young Joseph Fullwood, and John Carter senior, was another name for tin-plate working or tin smithing. A whitesmith was a worker in 'white iron' or tin, and was someone who polished or finished metal goods as distinguished from someone who forged them.

Other occupations and trades mentioned above are screw maker, rule maker, locksmith, iron brazier, wood-screw maker, stove-screw maker and seamstress. The high proportion of industrial metalworking occupations is indicative of Wolverhampton in the 19th century, which was rapidly becoming known as the lock-making centre of the region. Nail and screw making were also highly important trades in the town. The 1827 map, produced for Smart's Trade Directory of the same year, begins with a description of the town of Wolverhampton, noting its pre-eminence in the manufacture of every article 'in the ironmongery line and of goods of which brass, iron and steel are the component materials'. The author also notes that the former thriving trade in steel chains, buckles and sword hilts, etc, scarcely remained due to the French

Revolution, but that the loss had been partly offset by a rise in the production of tin, papier mâché and japanned wares. Like Birmingham, the town was involved in the production of metal goods from an early date, at least by the end of the 16th century, paralleling similar developments in other neighbouring places such as Walsall, Dudley and Halesowen. The production of such goods relied on a chain of different specialised manufacturers and finishers.

It is likely that the whitesmiths and screw makers etc worked from their homes or from workshops to the rear of their homes, although some may have been employed in the larger factories that were beginning to appear.

Charles Street, housing and health

Charles Street had been laid out by 1827, but was not extant in 1750 – at that time only the eastern part of the road existed, and was named Four Ashes. A public house known as the Four Ashes was still standing on Charles Street in the 1950s. To its south were gardens or allotments and, to the north, housing. Charles Street joined North Street with Stafford Street, two approximately parallel streets running north-south on the west and east sides of the town respectively. It also merged with High Street, at which angle lay the overflow St Peter's burial ground. Thus the Carters and Fullwoods were buried just around the corner from where they had lived.

An 1871 map shows terraced buildings along each side of Charles Street at its western end. At its eastern end are more irregularly spaced and shaped buildings. Plates 41–

77

43 show the type of terraced housing still extant in the 1950s, which may well have been standing for a century or more already. In 1875, the Artisans and Labourers Dwellings Act was passed and this led to the clearance of some of the worst slums. It is perhaps not surprising that John Carter died of phthisis and his son of diarrhoea given that Wolverhampton was known as a 'midden town', a town without any means of mains drainage. Housing consisted of back-to-backs and Dr Delane, reporting in the 1840s, states that the houses 'are themselves often of the very worst construction, and in immediate contact with extensive receptacles of manure and rubbish' (Upton 1998). The worst housing was in the north and east around Stafford Street, Walsall Street, Salop Street and Caribbee Island. As mentioned above, Charles Street joined Stafford Street with North Street and is likely to have suffered from the same poor standards.

Two cholera epidemics, in 1849 and 1857, may well have killed some of the children belonging to the families above, and a smallpox epidemic in 1871–2 claimed 483 lives. 1871 was the year that the young Thomas Watwood Carter died from diarrhoea.

CHAPTER 7

Discussion

Josephine Adams and Kevin Colls

The results of the excavations undertaken in the overflow burial ground of St Peter's Church, Wolverhampton, invite discussion of several key areas. The anthropological information has informed our understanding of the people who lived and died in Wolverhampton during the 19th century, allowing comparisons to be made with populations recorded in other post-medieval burial grounds. The examination of the burial practices has also provided an opportunity to compare and contrast funeral ritual in the town with that seen in contemporary burial grounds in the Midlands, revealing both similarities and differences in local traditions.

The study of the recovered skeletal assemblage from St Peter's has painted a general picture of the quality of life experienced by the individuals analysed, along with information regarding the nature of their deaths. Only one individual, James White (HB 70), was identified by the presence of a coffin plate – he is therefore the only individual within the skeletal assemblage with known sex, age at death and occupation. His age determination was not an easy task, because the morphological traits used to make the assessment gave an older biological age (46+) than the chronological age (42) obtained from the historical record. This overestimation in age is quite unusual; a study of the reliability of age determination methods carried out on evidence from Christ Church, Spitalfields, suggested that older skeletons tended to be under-aged and the young skeletons over-aged (Molleson *et al* 1993).

The human skeletal remains recovered from the excavation reveal a broad variety of pathological conditions that leave traits on the bone such as trauma, congenital and developmental anomalies, specific and non-specific infections, metabolic diseases, neoplastic conditions and joint-related diseases. In particular, in juveniles, diseases like rickets, scurvy, *cribra orbitalia*, growth retardation and dental enamel hypoplasia were recorded. It is during childhood when these stress indicators appear, as a result of poor diet and living conditions, leading to a high rate of child mortality. At St Peter's, over 40% of the individuals studied died before they were 18 years old.

During the 19th century, Wolverhampton experienced a rapid growth in both population and local industry, including mining and metalworking (Wohl 1983, 261). Skeletal analysis revealed many injuries and conditions which were likely to have been a result of occupation.

The growth of mechanisation and factory-based work resulted not only in trauma caused by machinery misuse but also injuries relating to repetitive movement (Roberts and Cox 2003). The high prevalence of OA and enthesopathies in the assemblage can be linked to some extent to occupational activities which would have involved stress to the joints. Most of the traumatic elements recorded, such as amputation, fracture, and *myositis ossificans traumatica* may also have been related to industrial accidents. The number of cases exhibiting ante mortem fractures in at least one bone was 18 individuals, which corresponds to 19.5% of the total adult population assessed. The study of trauma was characterised by a high frequency of rib fractures in both sexes – perhaps a consequence of domestic and/ or work-related accidents or even violent incidents. Two men (HB 56, HB 120) had well-healed fractures in some metacarpal bones. The latter was of particular note, since together with two healed fractures of the nose, he also had healed fractures of both thumbs and the right 1st and left 4th metacarpal. In a study by Brickley and Smith on similar fractures in the St Martin's assemblage it was concluded that this type of injury could have been caused by bare-knuckle boxing, a sport that was popular at the time. This style of fighting, in contrast to contemporary boxing techniques, involves the boxers holding their fists vertically to punch, resulting in more damage to the thumbs and 1st metacarpal (Brickley and Smith 2006, 173). The injuries to HB 120 could therefore indicate that he took part in this sport.

The three cases of amputation found in the assemblage were very interesting as they showed evidence of healing and survival after the operation as well as direct evidence for this medical procedure in Wolverhampton during the 19th century. One individual (HB 53) appeared to have had her left arm torn off, probably as a consequence of an accident rather than of it having been surgically amputated. As a result, the elbow joint was retained with two vestigial forms of ulna and radius, which appear to have formed a small stump below the joint. The other two individuals (HB 86 and HB 129) had had surgical amputations carried out. According to the rival schools of amputation during the first half of the 19th century, these individuals would have been subject to either a circular operation (also called *tour de maître*), which consisted of using a circular stroke to divide skin and muscles, or a 'flap operation' (Witkin 1997). The reasons why these amputations were carried out are unknown but it can be assumed that a life-threatening event such as severe infection, trauma, or cancer was the explanation

(Duckworth 1980). In general, such medical procedures were only affordable to wealthier people (Wood and Woodward 1984). However, it cannot be assumed that the aforementioned amputees were wealthy, since in 1821 a People's Dispensary had been established in Queen Street, adjacent to St Peter's, by wealthy local businessmen who were concerned about the health of the poor. One of the first patrons was Dr E H Coleman who, on January 1st 1847, performed a leg amputation on an 18-year-old girl. This was one of the first operations performed under general anaesthetic in England and the availability of this procedure could have been a contributory factor in the success of this and other operations in the town (Stallard undated 10).

The heavy industrial activity which may have given rise to the name 'Black Country' was also a contributing factor to people's general health. In his novel of 1841, *The Old Curiosity Shop*, Charles Dickens describes how the region's local factory chimneys 'poured out their plague of smoke, obscured the light, and made foul the melancholy air'. The 'plague' of smoke and other air pollution inevitably led to pulmonary diseases within the local population. One of the St Peter's individuals identified from a grave memorial (but not related to a burial), beer retailer John Carter, died of phthisis (tuberculosis), a pulmonary consumption related to damp conditions and air pollution. This disease spread significantly in the 19th century due to crowded environments, poor living conditions and an increase in the ingestion of dairy products. Consequently, tuberculosis became the principal cause of death in the Victorian period (Aufderheide and Rodríguez-Martín 1998, 130). Only one individual (HB 40) showed tuberculous lesions in the spine, providing osteological evidence of tuberculosis within the skeletal assemblage. However, the percentage of rib lesions (deposits of new bone on their visceral side) suggestive of long-standing and chronic infection may also represent a high prevalence of tuberculosis in the St Peter's group. It should not be forgotten, however, that rib lesions can also be produced by diseases such as chronic bronchitis and other pulmonary infections which were common in these industrial environments, due to the lack of good ventilation and a high quantity of smoke concentrated in both the living and working areas (Wohl 1983).

Another specific infection present in skeletal assemblage was syphilis. In total, there were two cases, one male (HB44) and one female (HB75), both middle-aged individuals. In the 19th century there was great discussion amongst the medical profession about the connection between insanity and syphilis. Certainly, in some cases, the final stages of the disease could result in dementia and violent physical fits (Quetel 1986, 162). Conjecture could then arise about the state of mind of the syphilitic male (HB 44) who had peri-mortem fractures of the humerus and tibia. The fracture of such large bones at or just prior to death could suggest a fairly violent demise.

The female (HB 75) had a thickened right tibia and fibula, which is compatible with the appearance of syphilis. It is not known whether HB 75 received any special treatment or hospital attention to alleviate her disease, although from the 16th century onwards syphilis was widely treated with mercury ointment (Aufderheide and Rodríguez-Martín 1998). The presence of mercury in another grave (HB 140) may highlight the availability and usage of this treatment during this time (Neilson and Coates 2002).

Three skeletons were identified with malignant neoplastic conditions, representing 3.2% of the assemblage. This rate is considerably higher than that seen at other contemporary sites, such as Christ Church, Spitalfields, (0.1%) and Redcross Way (0.68%) (Roberts and Cox 2003). One possible explanation for this is that the St Peter's assemblage included an elevated number of mature adults who contracted the malignant condition but lived long enough for it to affect the skeleton. One adult male (HB 39) exhibited well-preserved sunburst appearance on some vertebrae and ribs. Even though it was a dramatic case and its cause is unknown, it is possible to label it as an osteosarcoma. Alternatively, the degree of preservation of the bones themselves may account for the higher frequency.

Infant mortality at the site was very high, with 76% of juveniles having died before the age of five. In addition, it was possible to assess a sexual differentiation in the distribution of mortality of the adult population. The mortality rate in females was higher during the younger age categories, probably due to the risks of pregnancy and parturition. However, if they survived these risky periods, they enjoyed more longevity than males. As with any cemetery population, it is worth noting that many pathologies and conditions are likely to be underrepresented due to the 'osteological paradox'; if a disease or condition kills an individual quickly enough, no evidence will be identifiable on the bones.

THE WIDER CONTEXT: COMPARISONS

Skeletal analysis

The results of the skeletal analysis on the human remains excavated at St Peter's overflow burial ground have been compared to three other post-medieval burial sites: St Bartholomew's Church, Penn, Wolverhampton, St Martin's, Birmingham, and Holy Trinity in Coventry. In 2001, 857 burials were recorded during archaeological work at St Martin's Church in Birmingham (Brickley *et al* 2006). Similarly in 1999, 1706 burials were recorded during archaeological fieldwork in the overspill graveyard of Holy Trinity Church, Coventry (Soden and Wakeley, pers. comm.) and 372 burials were excavated during work at St Bartholomew's Church (Boyle 2004). Anthropological analysis of the skeletal remains, investigating demography and health, offers some marked differences when compared to St Peter's. It is important to note that only a sample number of skeletal remains

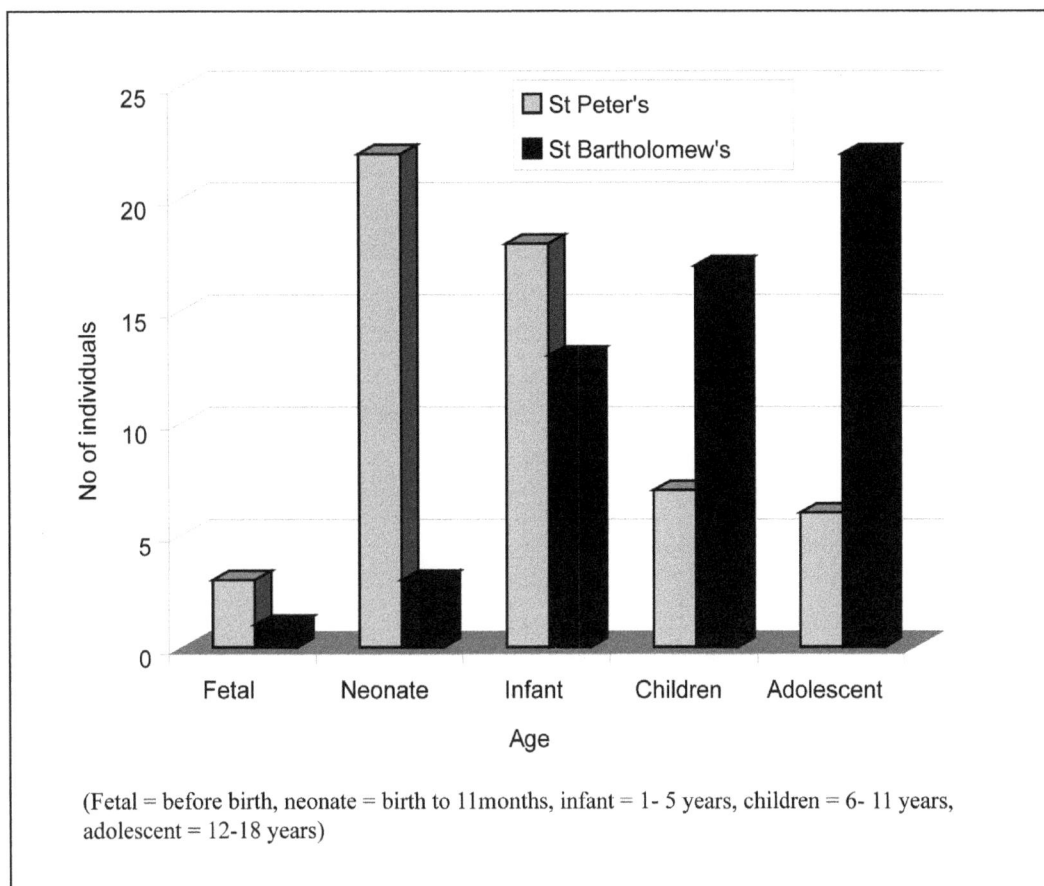

(Fetal = before birth, neonate = birth to 11months, infant = 1- 5 years, children = 6- 11 years, adolescent = 12-18 years)

Figure 17 Age breakdown of sub-adults from St Peter's and St Bartholomew's

from St Martin's and Holy Trinity were assessed, 505 and 100 respectively.

St Bartholomew's Church, Penn
Analysis of the human remains recovered from excavations at St Bartholomew's revealed that the sample population appeared to be a healthy one which lived well into old age (Boyle 2004). Some 84.4% of the individuals were adults (over the age of 18), with over half of these aged 40 and above. This is in contrast to St Peter's where 42% of the individuals died before the age of 20, with only 20% aged 46 years or over.

A breakdown of the age at death for the sub-adults from St Bartholomew's also highlights a marked difference to the St Peter's assemblage. As demonstrated in Fig 17, some 71% of the sub-adults from the Penn population died after the age of five. The opposite statistic is revealed from the St Peter's data set, where 76% of the sub-adults died before the age of five. These demographic profiles are somewhat typical when comparing rural and urban post-medieval burial sites. Evidence suggests that the populations of the out-of-town, or rural, cemeteries such as St Bartholomew's, were somewhat wealthier than the populations living within the urban centres. These 'middle class' areas would undoubtedly have been more privileged, particularly when considering factors which contribute to quality of life, such as health care, food,

housing, sanitation and even employment. Other evidence recovered from the fieldwork at Penn reinforces this hypothesis. Many of the coffin fittings were made of brass and not iron and the personal memorials suggested a pattern of affluence. One vault in particular consisted of an 'elaborate doorway arch' (Boyle 2004), again standing testament to the wealth of the occupiers.

A similar picture emerges when considering skeletal pathology. Although the pathological data is somewhat incomplete from St Bartholomew's, some interesting points can be identified. The majority of pathology identified was degenerative joint disease associated with old age (Boyle 2004). There were very few cases of individuals exhibiting trauma such as fractures – in contrast to that seen at St Peter's where one major contributing cause of such injuries is considered to have been work-related accidents. This may therefore suggest that the types of work undertaken by the people of Penn were less hazardous.

St Martin's Church and Holy Trinity Church.
As highlighted in Chapter 5, over 42% of the recorded burials from St Peter's contained sub-adult human remains, with peak mortality between six months and five years. Infant mortality is known to have been very high during this period and approximately 50% of individuals died before the age of 20 (Roberts and Cox 2003). As

St Peters

Old adult 20%
Fetal 2%
Infant 28%
Middle adult 22%
Children 7%
Young adult 16%
Adolescent 5%

St Martins

Fetal 2%
Old adult 24%
Infant 16%
Children 11%
Adolescent 4%
Middle adult 30%
Young adult 13%

Holy Trinity

Fetal 2%
Infant 9%
Old adult 44%
Children 12%
Adolescent 6%
Young adult 7%
Middle adult 20%

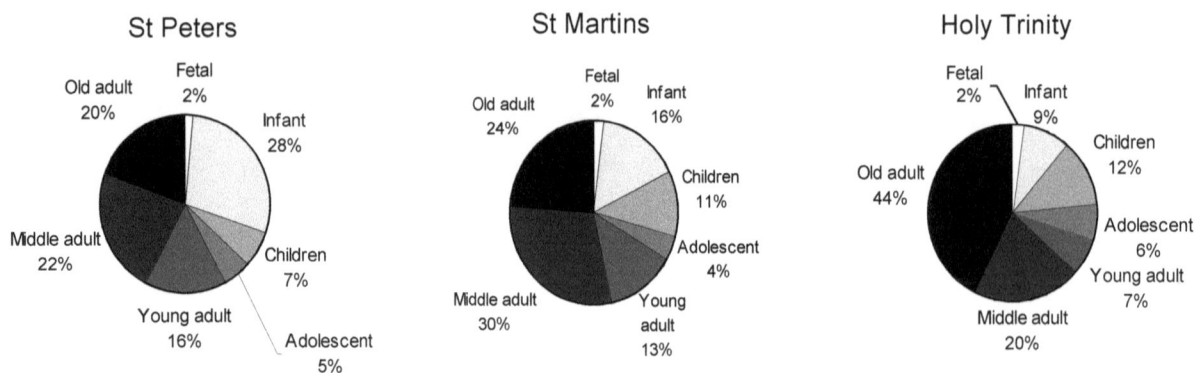

Fetal = before birth, infant = birth – 3 years, children = 3 – 12 years , adolescent = 12 – 20 years, young adult = 20 – 35 years, middle adult = 35 – 46 years, old adult = 46 years +

Figure 18 Age at death. Three burial ground populations compared

demonstrated in Fig 18, whilst the three study sites have a lower percentage of mortality before the age of 20 than is perhaps expected, there are a number of marked differences between the demographic profiles of each site.

The most marked difference is the high mortality rate of infants (birth to three years of age) buried at St Peter's. There is no doubt that death of newborns and young infants was frequent during this period. Inadequate weaning regimes led to deficient nutrition and an inability to fight diseases, viruses and infections, and although a high level of mortality amongst newborns has been documented from several other post-medieval cemetery sites, including St Martin's and Christ Church, Spitalfields (Molleson *et al* 1993), the 28% noted from St Peter's is especially high. Conversely, the infant mortality rate from Holy Trinity, Coventry, is especially low at 9%. This may suggest significant differences between the methods of nurturing newborns in Wolverhampton and in Coventry; however, given the small number studied at Coventry, it is difficult to draw such conclusions. The number of burials recovered during the excavation at St Peter's is only a small percentage of what would have been the entire population of the burial ground. It is therefore possible to theorise that at some time the small area of the burial ground covered as part of this study was used to bury newborns and infants. This would create a distorted demographic profile. Other than this high percentage of infant burials, the demographic profiles observed from St Peter's and St Martin's are indeed similar.

Another difference worthy of comment is the high percentage of older adult burials (46+ years old) recorded at Holy Trinity. This suggests that individuals from Coventry were living to an older age than their counterparts in either Wolverhampton or Birmingham. One possible explanation could be inferred when a comparison between the Victorian trade and industries in these towns was made. A visitor to 18th-century

Coventry would have encountered a large, populous city notable for its weaving and ribbon manufacture and watch-making and silk-weaving industry (Fox 1947). At its peak in 1857, the ribbon industry found employment for some 25,000 people. This is in contrast to Wolverhampton, as discussed in Chapter 2, where, by 1874, some 37,000 people (approximately 55% of the population) were employed as miners in the 469 collieries. This constituted a much more hazardous occupation for the workers, with accidents and fatalities being much more common. A similar picture becomes clear in Birmingham with small-scale industrial activities such as iron and steel manufacture and brass foundries constituting a high percentage of employment during the 19th century. Although simplistic, this evidence does suggest that the day-to-day work of the population of Coventry was, in general, much less labour intensive and certainly less hazardous. However, other contributory factors such as public health and diet should also considered and, given the fact that the Coventry sample is very small, substantial conclusions cannot be reached at this stage.

Health

A comparison of some of the pathologies and their crude prevalence rates was undertaken between the skeletal remains recovered from St Peter's and St Martin's. As the sites shared both a temporal and geographical framework, analysis was intended to highlight similarities and differences in the lifestyles of the two populations. The results are described in Chapter 5 and the implications considered below.

The skeletal remains recovered from both sites came from urban graveyards and represent a cross-section of the working classes of the earlier 19th century. The comparison of pathologies and health suggests that the way of life in the two population centres was basically the same. They shared similar environments, living conditions, culture, and problems. This is apparent when comparing the rates of stress indicator metabolic diseases such as *cribra orbitalia* and rickets, and some dental pathologies and neoplasia. In each case the frequency of these conditions in the two populations was similar. The living conditions were poor with houses badly overcrowded and often situated close to rubbish and compost heaps. The prevalence of enamel hypoplasia, another stress indicator, at the two sites is related to sex. At St Peter's the males were much more affected than the females, whereas the reverse was true at St Martin's. This suggests that the males from St Peter's and the females from St Martin's suffered more stress throughout their early life. This may be linked to employment, as boys in Wolverhampton would have began work in the mines at an early age, as would young girls in Birmingham in their role as domestic servants.

Despite the similarities in living conditions, some differences are apparent when the pathologies related to industrial activities/ work are analysed. These differences seems to be related to more risky occupational activities at St Peter's and differences between the sexes and the type of work performed. During the 19th century, mechanisation and factory working conditions produced not only trauma caused by the misuse of machinery but also injuries related to repetitive movements (Roberts and Cox 2003). The prevalence of OA and fractures at St Peter's can be linked in some extent to these occupational activities, like mining, which probably involved a lot of stress on the joints. At St Martin's, by contrast, the major cause for these pathological manifestations was age. These figures could imply that the occupational activities carried out by the population from St Peter's were more hazardous and more demanding physically than the ones at St Martin's, although as the demographic comparison above suggests, life expectancy was similar in both populations.

Furthermore, at St Martin's it is evident that some jobs were sex-related. For instance, a lot of the women were working as domestic servants. This work does not involve the risk or the mechanical stress that an industrial job would demand. This difference in occupation between the sexes at St Martin's is confirmed by the CPR results for *osteochondritis dissecans*. At St Martin's the males were more likely to be the victims of traumatic events such as industrial accidents.

Interestingly, the analysed sample from Holy Trinity in Coventry identified cases of traumas and fractures consistent with work-related accidents such as fractures of the hands and ribs and spinal injuries (Soden and Wakely, pers. comm.). However, these were far fewer in number than at the other two sites, supporting the hypothesis that the occupations undertaken in Coventry were less intensive and less hazardous than the types of employment in Wolverhampton or Birmingham.

Burial patterns at St Peter's Church
St Peter's Churchyard and its overflow burial ground have been the final resting place for many of

Wolverhampton's inhabitants since they were built. Parish burial records begin only 400 years ago and the church burial registers detail the number of people to have been buried in the grounds (see Chapter 2). In addition to knowing the numbers of burials from written records, and information pertaining to the health and demography of the population from skeletal remains, the actual location and pattern of these burials on the land within the church's jurisdiction provides a further point of discussion.

In common with other urban churches, and indeed some rural ones of the established church, a burial at St Peter's Church could take place in the church itself (intramural), the surrounding churchyard (extramural), or in an overflow burial ground. In this case it was the overflow burial ground of St Peter's that was excavated. The incidence of small burial grounds detached from churches was not uncommon. In Edinburgh, as early as 1718 the Old Calton Burying-Ground was opened, and in London between 1800 and 1830 15 small burial grounds were created to address the problem of overcrowding. These burial grounds were often surrounded by high walls to provide security against the grave robber (Curl 2000, 34– 55). They are described by Charles Dickens in *The Uncommercial Traveller* as '…churchyards sometimes so entirely detached from churches, always so pressed upon by houses; so small, so rank, so silent, so forgotton, except by the few people who ever look down into them from their smoky windows' (Dickens 1933, 676). Direct parallels can be drawn here between the St Peter's overflow burial ground and St Martin's in Birmingham. St Martin's, also an urban church, had both intramural and extramural burials and an overflow burial ground in nearby Park Street. These two are then compared to St Bartholomew's Church in Penn, a small rural village two miles to the southwest of Wolverhampton where both churchyard and vault burials took place.

An intramural burial, that is a burial in a church, was a high-status location and for centuries was considered the ultimate honour, reserved initially for monarchs, high-ranking clergy, founders and church benefactors. However, the realisation that prestigious plots in a church could command high returns led churches like St Peter's to extend the privilege to local wealthy people who looked to their parish church for a final resting place for themselves and their families (Litten 1991, 199). At St Peter's, this practise is illustrated by James Leveson, a local wool merchant and his family who have a tomb in the chapel, while the north side of the church has been traditionally used by the people of Willenhall, notably the Lane family who supported Charles II during the Civil War (Mander and Tildesley 1960, 179).

Burial outside the church in the land immediately around the building (extramural) was, for many, the obvious choice, but this, too, was often an indicator of wealth and social status as there were different options available. In the 18th and 19th centuries, when the number of burials at St Peter's was highest, the town of Wolverhampton was a growing industrial area (see Chapter 2). The majority of burials would have been from the working classes for whom the cost of an elaborate funeral may have been a serious consideration. For many, the only choice open to them was burial in an earth-cut grave, the cheapest option available, whilst others with slightly more disposable income may have opted for burial in a brick-lined grave.

For those of a higher social standing, like the wealthier landowners or mine owners, however, without the option of a intramural burial (either because of space constraints or because they were not considered of a high enough status), the alternative of burial in a vault in the churchyard was the next most favourable option. However, this too could be graded within the churchyard, with the wealthy wanting to buy vaults in the most attractive parts of the burial ground (Jalland 1996, 215).

If people were of a lower social status or were unable to afford the luxury of a vault, the next alternative was to purchase a brick-lined grave. This in itself indicated some degree of social standing and provided some additional security. The burial records indicate that brick-lined graves were built in both the churchyard and the burial ground, although none were revealed by the excavation. Finally the earth-cut grave was the remaining option for the majority of people.

The location of the grave was sometimes important to indicate status since the proximity to the church could have been another indicator of the social status of the burial (Adams 2006, 16). This burial ground at St Peter's had been built after the main churchyard had become overcrowded, in the same way as the Park Street burial ground had been opened to ease the pressure on St Martin's. Subsequently, the Park Street burial ground became known as a very undesirable location '...as only fit for the poorest of the poor...and was well called the "black spot" of the town' (Showell's *Dictionary of Birmingham* 1885, 32). Likewise the state of St Peter's burial ground became a source of public concern, as it too became overcrowded and neglected. It may have been considered a less desirable place to be buried and left for those without the means or the status to be buried next to the church.

It is impossible to speculate on the numbers buried in the new burial ground because, in a similar way to the burial records at St Martin's, the actual location of the burial at St Peter's (ie in the original churchyard or in the new burial ground) is not generally specified, apart from a five-year period between June 1850 and July 1855. During this time the churchwarden added more detail to the burial register and, whilst this only relates to a short time, it does allow some tentative conclusions to be drawn about the burial patterns in the churchyard and burial ground. Table 62 illustrates that many people recorded as buried at St Peter's after 1850 were in fact

Table 62 The location of the burials between June 1850 and July 1855

No. of burials 1850-1855	155
Cemetery (Merridale)	47
Vault in churchyard	23
Vault in new ground	27
Vault (unspecified)	4
New burial ground	16
Churchyard	6
Brick grave in old churchyard	2
Brick grave in new ground	5

NB The location of the remaining burials on this list is unspecified

interred at the new cemetery, having had their funeral service at the church. It is likely that this figure increased over the ensuing years as the cemetery became the main place of burial in the town. It would seem that the burial registers become a record of funerals rather than of burials, making it even more difficult to deduce the numbers of people buried in the grounds of the church.

The table also shows that some burials were still taking place in vaults in both the old and new burial grounds. Amongst the list, Samuel Lloyd is described in 1850 as being buried in a new vault. This indicates that at that time vaults were still being built, although whether it was in the churchyard or burial ground is unspecified. However, it is probable that it was in the latter, since space would have been at a premium in the churchyard and vault burials there would have been the preserve of those families who had existing vaults.

Whilst it is not possible to make a direct comparison of all this information with the vault burials at St Martin's, because those were extramural burials in a churchyard rather than an overflow burial ground (the direct comparison of this site would be with the Park Street burial ground), it is possible to compare those vault burials in the churchyard.

One notable difference provided by the burial records (although not revealed by the excavation) is that people of all ages, from as young as two months, were buried in the churchyard vaults at St Peter's whereas at St Martin's there was little documentary evidence of young babies. This could be accounted for by the fact that the vaults in Birmingham were bought by older more established families or by the fact that infants may have been buried elsewhere in the churchyard.

The occupants of the vaults at St Peter's, during this five-year period, were all local, apart from Mary Ann Cooper who died in 1851 and was listed as living in Southampton, and William Peace who died in 1852 in Leamington. The fact that they were brought back to Wolverhampton to be buried suggests that both families may have had a family vault, and sufficient means to pay for the considerable costs of transporting them back. This need to be buried with the rest of the family was also indicated in the St Martin's vaults where several people were brought back to the family vault from other towns. Similarly, at St Martin's, one of the vault burials died in Leamington and another lady owned property in town when she died, suggesting that perhaps residence in the nearby spa town was an aspiration of the middle classes (Adams in Brickley *et al* 2006, 195 and 208).

Amongst the 50 surnames on this part of the register that were described as buried in a vault, in either the churchyard or the burial ground, there were only a few that recurred, suggesting ownership of a family vault. The variety of the remaining names would seem to suggest that if people had requested a vault burial they may have been interred wherever there was a space. Thus the vaults, especially in the burial ground, may be considered more of a public rather than a private facility. As late as 1906, when Emma Humphryson was buried, a note was added stating that the vault was full, substantiating this theory.

It is unfortunate that the churchwardens did not continue with this extra information but this information over a five-year period does give some indication of the burial patterns.

By the late 1840s the burial ground was also becoming overcrowded and in 1850 a new cemetery opened in the town (see Chapter 2). This too has a parallel with other towns where it became fashionable to be buried in the new pleasant surroundings of the cemetery rather than the overcrowded churchyard. It is likely that the same choices of earth-cut, brick-lined or vault burials existed in the cemetery, but that is beyond the remit of this study. In Birmingham, where similar problems existed in the churchyards and burial grounds, Warstone Lane Cemetery had opened just two years before in 1848, providing its Anglican churches with an alternative burial place, and likewise in Kensal Green in London in 1833 and in Liverpool in 1825 (Curl 2000, 135).

Vaults

A vault could be one of two types. Either a 'family' vault, bought by those wealthy enough to be able to purchase a vault for members of their own family, or a parish vault, provided by the church to accommodate those who wanted a vault burial but could not afford a family vault. Initially, vaults were built in the churchyard as close to the church as possible and at St Peter's this could relate to the vaults in the original churchyard built in the late 18th century (see Chapter 2). The parish records list 21 occupants of these vaults along the west side of the churchyard associated with names and dates between 1774 and 1797. Two of those listed were clergymen of the church suggesting that at least some of them were used by local dignitaries. In 1834, the curate, a Dr Oliver, was responsible for building more vaults in the churchyard (see Chapter 2). It is not known for whom

these were built, but he may well have been responding to local demand. If these were indeed parish vaults built by the church, in the same way as a large vault at St Martin's (Brickley *et al* 2006), they may have provided a source of income for the church.

The vaults that were excavated were in the overflow ground. They could have been built there because the ground around the church was full, or they could have been the aforementioned parish vaults. The occupants that were identified, although relatively well off, were not drawn from the upper classes. There were other unidentified burials in the vaults, so it is not possible to say whether the vaults were built for one specific family or not.

Skeletal analysis of the burials in Vault 7 reveals that all six reached adulthood, with all but two being over the age of 36. This would suggest that these people had a better quality of life and therefore lived longer than many others in the burial ground population. This could be attributed to such factors as healthier diets, improved living conditions and access to medical treatment. One particular individual (HB 53) survived a traumatic amputation and lived for many years afterwards, which suggests that she was able to afford expensive high quality medical care. The tentative conclusion could be drawn therefore, that the individuals recovered from Vault 7 were wealthier, and therefore able to afford to purchase space in a vault.

The reasons for wanting a vault burial were complex. The increasing importance of the family in the newly emerging, 19th-century middle classes perhaps provides one reason. The home was seen as a place of sanctuary, separate from the husband's work, a place that he could return to at the end of the day and enjoy the company of his wife and family (Davidoff and Hall 1994, 364–9). Likewise, the family vault united the family in death as in life, and separated them from the working classes buried in ordinary graves in the churchyard.

In addition, for the *nouveaux riches* of Wolverhampton, it was a way to demonstrate their success in life. As well as the trappings of the funeral, the final resting place was the subject of much consideration, and one that could make a very public statement about one's social worth. Amongst the vaults in the churchyard were those belonging to the Mander family on the north side of the church, a family that for generations had contributed to the life of the town, the Holland vault along the drive, and the Blackhurst vault on the south side.

It has been argued that another pertinent factor was the growth of the medical profession. To satisfy the growing demand for medical teaching a large supply of corpses was constantly needed for anatomy tuition. The only legal source was the gallows, so some enterprising individuals looked to the overcrowded urban graveyards for an easy source of fresh corpses. These grave robbers, or 'resurrectionists' as they were called, became the source of great fear and hatred, as the violation of the grave was abhorred at all levels of society (Richardson 1987, 108). This fear resulted in stringent methods being introduced to thwart the robbers, special iron coffins with locks, coffin screws that could not be loosened, iron railings, and even straw placed over a coffin lengthways and crossways between layers of earth over the coffin to hinder any subsequent excavation. This latter practice has been noted at nearby St Paul's in Birmingham (McKenna 1992, 17). Another means of security was, of course, the deep grave or secure vault. Whilst there is no evidence of a resurrectionist threat at Wolverhampton, there was an anatomy school in Birmingham in 1828 that would have needed a constant supply of corpses. Since the practice of grave robbing did not cease until the Anatomy Act was passed in 1832, it is possible therefore that the fear of grave robbing stimulated some people in Wolverhampton to consider the security of a vault (Richardson 1987, 88).

Vault construction
In general, vaults did not have a strict pattern of construction. Some were rendered or lime washed, others left as plain brick. Some had drainage or ventilation and others had an internal charnel pit. However, the vaults at St Peter's were similar in construction to some of the intramural vaults excavated at St Augustine the Less, Bristol (Boore 1998, 71). They were all designed in the same way, rectangular in shape with red brick walls and barrel-vaulted brick roofs, and lime washed inside. The brick floors were bedded in sand, either in parallel rows or in a herringbone pattern. One vault on the Bristol site had one face with alternate niches giving a dovecote effect similar to that seen in Vault 3. Boore suggests that this may have had some personal significance for the occupant of the vault or may have simply been due to a shortage of bricks. The similarity between sites suggests that in some cases there was little difference between intramural and extramural vault construction.

As Vaults 1 to 6 were so similar in design and construction the suggestion is that they were all built at the same time, and burial places sold to families who wanted to be buried in a vault. They may have been built by the church to fulfil local needs, while also raising parish funds. At St Martin's, a larger vault housing different families was built by the church for those who could not afford an individual family vault, and there may be a parallel here with Vault 7 that was built further away from the others (Brickley *et al* 2006). Another reason why Vault 7 was built away from the others could be attributed to a local rumour that smallpox victims from the General Hospital were placed there during the epidemic in the 1870s, although no documentary evidence exists to support this (G Bolton, pers. comm.).

The vaults here were small in comparison to those at St Martin's that were mostly rectangular in shape and cut into or to the top of the natural sandstone. Features of the vaults at St Martins also included whitewashed interior

walls, internal divisions made of brick, and barrel-vaulted roofs (Buteux & Cherrington in Brickley *et al* 2006, 29–30). The interior of the vaults sometimes contained shelves or local space for storage of the coffins. However, this was not the case at St Peter's where the vaults were too small for shelving or recesses, but Vaults 3, 5 and 6 (Figs 8 and 9) did show evidence of division into chambers. The size of the chambers varied and was not a simple division of the vault into two equal halves. The narrow chamber in Vault 6 presumably represented the outline of a smaller coffin deposited in the vault, with the dividing brick shouldering the coffin. It is likely that once the lower layer of the vault had been filled (probably only two adult coffins would fit the space) then a layer of slabs would provide a surface on which to place the next layer. Vaults 1, 2 and 4 did not contain any evidence of internal divisions, but this may have been destroyed during the 1973 clearance. Vault 7, although it showed no evidence of internal division, did contain six sets of remains, so the coffins may have been stacked on top of each other or supported by wooden coffin supports which had subsequently rotted away.

The vaults at St Peter's are similar in construction to those excavated at St Bartholomew's Church in Penn. The vaults here were built over a similar time span to St Peter's and display many of the same characteristics. The vaults are brick built with barrelled roofs and whitewashed walls, although some have more internal divisions, candle-holders and one a more elaborate entrance, suggesting perhaps higher status burials. An excavation at Tallow Hill Cemetery in Worcester, 59 kilometres away from Wolverhampton, also revealed vaults built in a similar style (Ogden *et al* 2005).

Earth-cut graves
The burials excavated here represent typical Church of England burials, in that the skeletons were found in an extended, supine position, deposited in coffins and aligned east-west. The excavation revealed many burials inter-cutting each other, and frequently there was evidence of more than one body in a grave cut (Plate 7). It was clear that the area had been filled as densely as possible to maximise use of the space available. In some churchyards it may be possible to recognise families interred together within specific parts of a burial ground or within a vault (O'Brien and Roberts 1996, 159), but in this case the high levels of truncation and partial clearance of the site made this impossible.

There were no brick-lined graves excavated although information from the burial register (see above) indicates that some had been built. Their absence could be due to a previous clearance on the site (see Chapter 2).

There were few grave goods, but those that were found were items from clothing, or jewellery, which were probably from the burial outfit or last garment worn rather than deliberately placed in the grave. A button or stud was found with HB 63. This was an infant of 0–3 months so it may have been from the clothing of a person who cared for, or buried, the child (see Bevan, Chapter 4).

An almost complete china cup (SF3) was found with HB 25 (Plate 14). This could have been a favourite item of the deceased or something that grieving relatives most associated with the person. A French custom involved a ceramic drinking vessel or stoup filled with holy water that was kept by the coffin prior to interment and then thrown into the grave on top of the coffin and buried with it. This may originally have been a Catholic tradition absorbed into English culture following the Reformation (Cox 1998, 117). This may be one explanation for the presence of the cup, but it should also be remembered that, as the grave cuts were not clear, the cup might have been a result of later disturbance rather than deliberate deposition.

A metal ring on the chest of HB 42 may have been the remains of a wreath placed on the coffin. Floral tributes did not become fashionable until the 1860s (Litten 1991, 170) and that corresponds with the possible dates of the later burials within the family vaults. Wreaths were expensive so this was another indicator of wealth or an aspiration of the wealth of the occupants of the vault.

In Vault 6 a set of dentures was discovered (see Chapter 3). They could not be associated with a particular burial so the sex and status of the owner is impossible to establish. It is possible, however, using documentary sources to understand something of the culture of the day that necessitated the purchase of a set of false teeth.

The dentures available initially were not very effective for chewing food so the motive for wearing them depended more upon appearances. There was a difference here, though, between men and women, with the former not minding about taking their teeth out at mealtimes while the latter avoided it. This, together with the fear of their teeth slipping, explained why many Victorian women ate their sandwiches in their bedroom before dinner. This prevented the possible dental *faux pas* during the meal and also gave the favourable impression that Victorian women had small dainty appetites. The men, however, whilst not minding about eating without their dentures in, replaced them to improve their clarity of speech over the port! Unfortunately the spirit had a damaging effect on the ivory teeth and after about a year these became blackened and spoiled (Woodforde 1995, 65).

The state of a person's teeth also discouraged audible laughter for fear of displaying bad or missing teeth, or an inadequate replacement set. During the early 19th century ladies held a fan over their mouth in an attempt to mask the problem. However, by the end of the century, improvements in the manufacture of false teeth meant they no longer had to be hidden (Woodforde 1995, 28).

In the 1830s the idea of suction plates was muted to keep the dentures in place but it was not until the 1860s and 1870s that this was widely advertised. Even then, they did not always work and often failed at mealtimes, causing much embarrassment. The use of springs to keep the dentures in place, as in the set found here and on a more expensive set recovered from St Martin's Churchyard, must have been uncomfortable to wear and they often broke. A Victorian lady may often have had two pairs of teeth to avoid embarrassment in company. In addition, they had to be adjusted frequently as the gums began to shrink or else they became unstable and difficult to keep in place (Woodforde 1995, 68–9).

The owner of these dentures must have had sufficient means to pay for them, as well as considerable tooth decay to warrant the need for them. They may well have bought them from Mr De Loude, a Surgeon-Dentist in St John's Square who in 1838 advertised in Bridgens Directory of the Borough of Wolverhampton that he could make '…artificial teeth of every description, from a single tooth to a whole set' (see Fig 19).

One specific burial worthy of note was HB 140, which contained mercury beneath the *depositum* plate, in the abdominal region. Mercury can have serious side-effects and if taken in large quantities can be fatal. Accidental poisonings were fairly common in the 18th and presumably 19th centuries, and assuming that the mercury found associated with HB 140 was not later contamination, the amount found constituted a large dose and could have been the cause of death.

Whilst it was noted at Christ Church, Spitalfields, that syphilis was treated using mercury ointments, the mercury was detected in the bone material and not within the burial (Molleson *et al* 1993, 85). However, no further analysis of HB 140 was possible because the mercury had to be disposed of as contaminated waste. There were two possible cases of syphilis discovered on the site (HB 44 and HB 75: Chapter 5), but neither had evidence of any treatment involving mercury. The other known association with mercury and burials was found at 36 Craven Street, London, during excavation in 1997. A pit with the remains of humans and animals was found and was believed to have been the remains of the work of William Hewson from the late 18th century. Hewson was a student and partner of the anatomist William Hunter and best remembered for demonstrating the lymphatic system of the turtle using mercury. Turtle remains were found at Craven Street during the excavations (Hillson *et al* 1999). Whilst this is a tenuous suggestion concerning HB 140, it may be possible that during the mid-19th century a similar demonstration or process was carried out on a human.

A somewhat more plausible explanation for the presence of the mercury droplets in the stomach region of HB 140 may lie with the homeopathic remedy *Mercurius vivus*. This was a common remedy from the 18th century

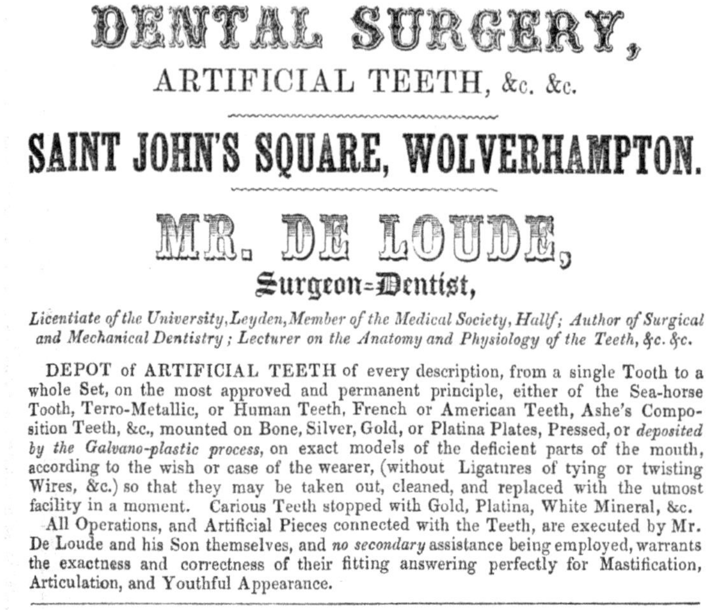

DENTAL SURGERY,
ARTIFICIAL TEETH, &c. &c.

SAINT JOHN'S SQUARE, WOLVERHAMPTON.

MR. DE LOUDE,
Surgeon-Dentist,

Licentiate of the University, Leyden, Member of the Medical Society, Hallf; Author of Surgical and Mechanical Dentistry; Lecturer on the Anatomy and Physiology of the Teeth, &c. &c.

DEPOT of ARTIFICIAL TEETH of every description, from a single Tooth to a whole Set, on the most approved and permanent principle, either of the Sea-horse Tooth, Terro-Metallic, or Human Teeth, French or American Teeth, Ashe's Composition Teeth, &c., mounted on Bone, Silver, Gold, or Platina Plates, Pressed, or *deposited by the Galvano-plastic process*, on exact models of the deficient parts of the month, according to the wish or case of the wearer, (without Ligatures of tying or twisting Wires, &c.) so that they may be taken out, cleaned, and replaced with the utmost facility in a moment. Carious Teeth stopped with Gold, Platina, White Mineral, &c.

All Operations, and Artificial Pieces connected with the Teeth, are executed by Mr. De Loude and his Son themselves, and *no secondary* assistance being employed, warrants the exactness and correctness of their fitting answering perfectly for Mastification, Articulation, and Youthful Appearance.

Figure 19 Advertisement in Bridgen's Directory of the Borough of Wolverhampton 1838

onwards and could be taken in both tablet and liquid form (Krapp and Longe c 2001: *Gale Encyclopedia of Alternative Medicine*). It has been used since ancient times to treat, amongst other things, fever, skin disorders, chickenpox, diarrhoea, and toothache. It is perhaps interesting to note that John Mander, one of the brothers who founded the very successful paint and varnish business in the town, also produced chemicals, including mercurial preparations for use in medicine and the arts (Mander and Tildesley 1960, 146). One could imagine that some sort of industrial accident could have taken place, but there is no real basis for such speculation. Another possible reason for the presence of mercury within the burial may be that the deceased was buried with an object containing mercury, for example a thermometer, however no evidence of any such object was found.

Contemporary burial practices and the local funeral industry

In the early 19th century the people of Wolverhampton would have been familiar with death. The increasing industrialisation that was transforming their lives was also contributing to the high mortality rates as the growing town failed to cope with the rise in population and increasingly unsanitary conditions. Work in the nearby mines was difficult and dangerous, while life in the overcrowded streets, with its mixture of workshop and home, contributed to the unhealthy lifestyle. Families were often large, but the deaths of infants and young children were a common fact of life that affected people of all classes, to different degrees (Jalland 1996, 120). Many parents lost many or all of their children (Brickley *at al* 2006), with diarrhoea, pneumonia, bronchitis and convulsions being the worst enemy in their first year, while measles, whooping cough and scarlet fever were

more dangerous after their first birthday. In Wolverhampton, there was the added danger of smallpox and cholera outbreaks (Chapter 2).

How people coped with this everyday occurrence is impossible to quantify. Amongst some of the middle classes religion was a fundamental part of their family life, providing structure to their lives, and within this framework some 'were brought up to remember that death was an essential part of life, and must be faced without fear' (Haldene in Jalland 1996, 3). It is possible that some of the working classes felt the same way, but apart from the emotional loss, the death of the family breadwinner could have been catastrophic. Conversely, the death of a child, whilst sad for many, for others might represent one less mouth to feed. In Wolverhampton, there is evidence to suggest that a higher proportion of the population attended a place of worship than in similar industrial centres (Chapter 2) but whether this helped them cope with the ever-present fear of death is unknown. It could be argued, however, that the ritual of the funeral helped people come to terms with the death, providing a structure for the grieving relatives and reuniting family groups. Amongst the middle and upper classes, where the ethos of the family was strongest, the rise of both the Evangelical and Romantic movements in the early 19th century encouraged people to express their feelings of grief at the death of a loved one (Jalland 1996, 12). In many cases this manifested itself in a very public way with the provision of a lavish funeral.

The reasons for the growing importance of the funeral were complex. The emerging middle classes, those who were starting to benefit from the profits of industrialisation, were beginning to display the fruits of their success. This was apparent not only in their houses, clothes and lifestyle but in pomp and ceremony surrounding their funeral. A successful businessman would have expected his death to demonstrate his success in life, and the archetypal view of the Victorian funeral of such a person is of a large black hearse with glass sides, drawn by six black horses adorned with black ostrich plumes. The coffin may have been lined with lead, and be made of oak or elm, lined with white satin, with expensive brass handles and engraved plates, and be draped with black or purple cloth. Behind the hearse would come the coaches with mourners in strict order of importance, all dressed in heavy black mourning. The men wore black bands of crape around their top hats, while the women were hidden by yards of black crape, used black-edged handkerchiefs, and wore black gloves. There were strict codes of etiquette to be followed for women, in particular, whose attire depended upon their relationship to the deceased, and the length of time since the death had occurred. This included the dress, but shawls, bonnets, veils, caps, umbrellas, and even the underwear were trimmed in black ribbon (Flanders 2003, 343–5; Curl 1972, 2–15). To satisfy this demand for a range of clothing and to ensure that the wealthy could buy all they needed from one place, specific shops opened exclusively for the sale of mourning costume and accessories. The Birmingham Mourning and Funeral Warehouse of Bach & Barker advertised in the Wolverhampton directories, suggesting that the wealthy people of the town would have to travel there to satisfy their need for outward respectability at a time of bereavement. Despite the need to be correctly dressed following a family bereavement, women did not usually attend upper and middle class funerals, on the grounds that they would be unable to control their feelings (Jalland 1996, 221). However, opinion was divided on this and advice in *Cassell's Household Guide* on funeral customs suggests that:

…there is no reason why women should not share it as well as men, always supposing that they can restrain their feelings. If there is any fear of their not being able to do this, they are much better at home. Private feeling and public grief should not be displayed in public, and the solemnity of the service for the dead should not be disturbed by an exhibition of the sorrow of the living (*Cassell's Domestic Dictionary* 1884).

In the same volume it is suggested that '…the window blinds are usually drawn down as soon as there has been a death in the house, and they are kept down until the funeral has left, when they are drawn up', indicating to the immediate community that a death has occurred. Subsequently some families would send out black-edged mourning cards that were often decorated in elaborate fashion, inviting selected people to attend the funeral. Other ostentatious displays might include hiring 'mutes', two men who wore frock coats and top hats and who, on the day of the funeral, stood either side of the front door of the house where the deceased lived. They carried crape-covered wands and were considered symbolic of

the visitation of death, and often walked alongside the hearse as it was drawn along the streets. After the ceremony a feast was provided for the mourners, an event which itself became a competition as neighbours vied with each other to provide the best fare. The food traditionally would include sherry, ham, pies, port with cakes, jelly and trifle. In some counties this feast was held before the burial with the body available for viewing, a custom said to have originated to ensure the corpse was actually dead (Curl 1972, 2–15).

In early 19th-century Wolverhampton it is likely that the richer members of local society had funerals similar to those described above. Indeed it is suggested that in Wolverhampton such was the public interest in funerals that when a member of the Royal Family died the newspaper of the day would devote whole pages with blackened borders to describe the scenes of the funeral and lying in state, spreading the details over several days to heighten the effect (Mander and Tildesley 1960, 159).

As the growing numbers of the middle class began to copy the gentry in their funerary customs, this social competition spread and the working classes, too, felt the need to emulate their superiors. For many, the fear of a parish funeral was akin to the social stigma of being in a workhouse in life, and the wish for a 'good funeral' was one of the strongest feelings amongst many of the working classes. They too wanted to demonstrate respectability, even if the costs of the event led them into even greater debt. This desire was encouraged by the advent of the 'burial club', to which members paid a regular amount to cover the cost of a decent funeral. These clubs, however, had no system of regulation and were often corrupt; some were run by unscrupulous undertakers who charged exorbitant fees to satisfy people's desire for respectability (Morley 1971, 25). Working-class women would have been unable to frequent the elegant funeral warehouse, but instead would have relied either upon mourning dress being passed on by neighbours or upon utilising local dyers whose livelihood depended upon their ability to dye customers' clothes as quickly as possible in time for the funeral (Flanders 2003, 341).

The people of the parish of St Peter's would have been used to seeing funerals almost daily, as the people of the town took their loved ones to be buried at the local church, either in the churchyard around the church or, when that was full, in the overflow burial ground near by. This public display served to advertise the whole occasion and the funeral became an increasingly complex ritual that was to become a significant part of people's lives, while also encouraging the growth of the lucrative funeral industry.

In Wolverhampton, documentary evidence suggests that the funeral industry was not as well developed as in nearby Birmingham. During the 1832 cholera outbreak in nearby Bilston such was the demand for coffins that the

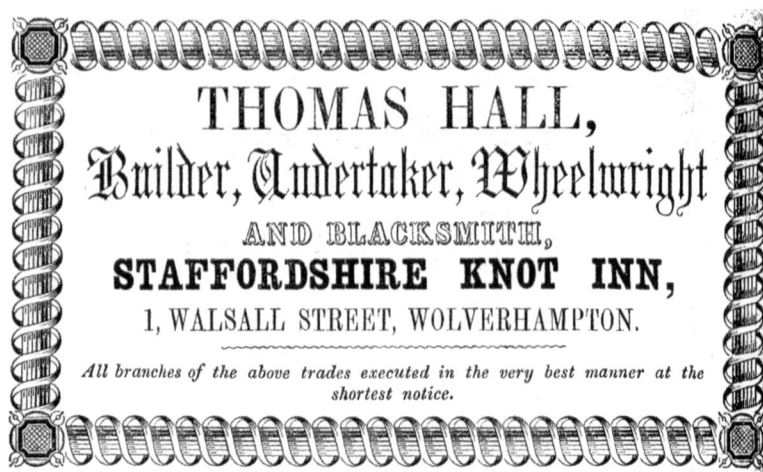

Figure 20 Advertisement from Post Office Directory of 1845: Thomas Hall

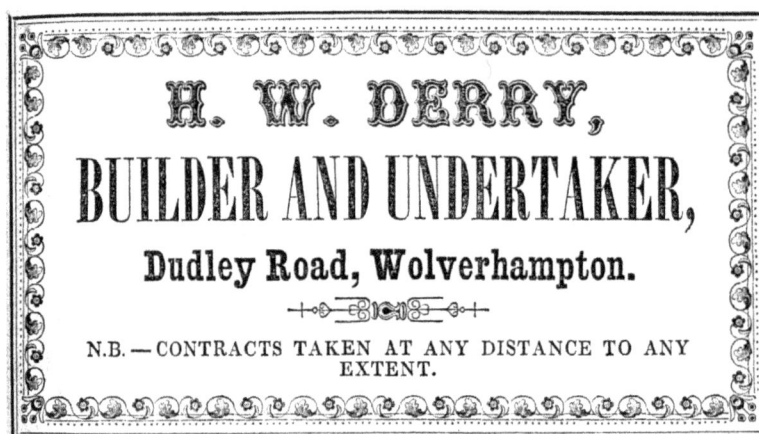

Figure 21 Advertisement from Post Office Directory of 1845: H W Derry

local firms could not cope '…so loads were brought in from Birmingham in open carts – without any covering' (Price 1832, 15).

In 1839, J Davis of New Road is listed in a local directory as a coffin maker. The manufacture of coffins was often undertaken by carpenters or upholsterers who were just looking to supplement their income, rather than relying on it to make a living. In contrast, George Jennings, another local carpenter, became something of a local entrepreneur, much in the spirit of the time. After conducting a funeral for a friend, he started an undertaking business that was to flourish until the present day, with the fifth generation of the family in charge (www.localhistory.scit.wlv.ac.uk/articles/Jennings). The wood used by these carpenters in the coffins at St Peters' was predominantly oak and elm with some pine, a similar selection to that found at St Martin's Church in Birmingham (Gale in Brickley *et al* 2006), although some spruce was also found (see Chapter 4).

The Post Office Directory of 1845 lists Paul Law at the Railway Hotel posting house operating Hearses and Mourning Coaches 'in constant readiness'. In 1851 Thomas Hall of 1 Walsall Street, Wolverhampton, was

advertised as a Builder, Undertaker and Wheelwright, while H W Derry was a Builder and Undertaker in Dudley Road (Figs 20 and 21). All of which demonstrate a degree of diversity that suggests they did not make their money from undertaking alone.

No evidence has been found to suggest that coffin furniture was made in the area although it is probable that somewhere amidst the many small metalworking workshops it was produced. However, following the excavation of the churchyard in the nearby village of Penn, the suggestion made there was that the coffin furniture was made in nearby Birmingham (Boyle 2004).

Two local businessmen who did capitalise on the demand for a respectable funeral were Mr Copage of the New Hotel, Cock Street, and Mr R Smith of Queen Street who advertised their 'Patent Funeral Carriage' (Fig 22). This aimed to bridge the gap between those who could only afford to walk behind the carriage to the churchyard and those who had the whole procession, by providing a carriage drawn by one horse that could hold both the coffin and the mourners, albeit 'quite separate and distinct'.

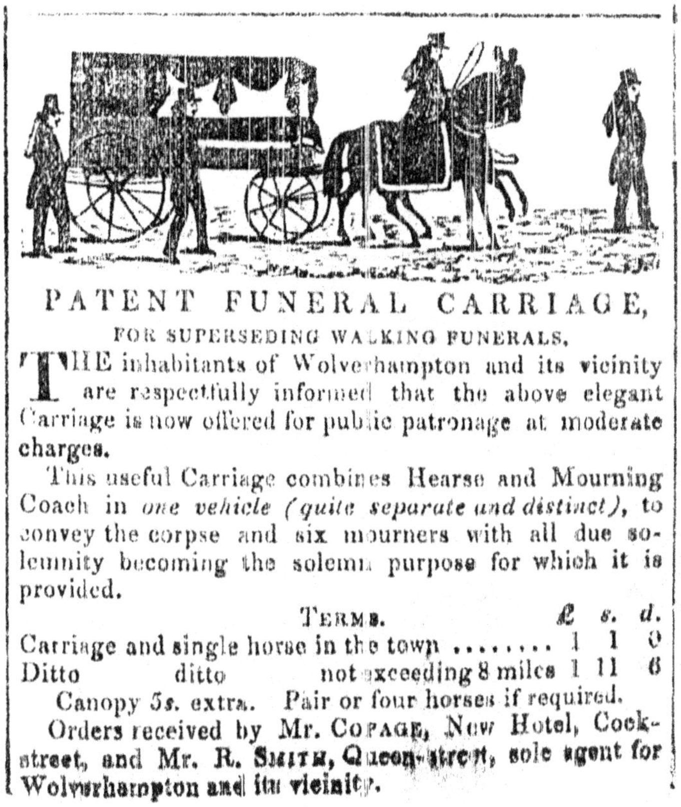

Figure 22 Advertisement for *Patent Funeral Carriage*

The people buried in the overflow burial ground

It is impossible to know precise detail about the people of Wolverhampton that were buried in this overflow burial ground. The parish records list only names, and during this excavation of a small part of it only one *depositum* plate that could be associated with a burial and several grave memorial stones were found. The plate provided insufficient detail for further research but the grave memorials produced information about four families (see Chapter 6).

In 1853, in an effort to address the problem of the overcrowded unsanitary urban burial ground, the government had passed the Metropolitan Interment Act (Jalland 1996, 199). This restricted burial in churchyards unless vault space was available, which suggests that any burial in the St Peter's records after this date must have been in a vault or existing family grave.

The dates on the grave memorials of the Carter and Fullwood family list dates of death in the 1860s and 1870s, indicative of a vault burial, so their presence associated with the excavated vaults could suggest they had purchased the vault for the use of their family. As in the case of St Martin's, the vault could have been purchased in anticipation of future bereavements, or at the time of death of a previous member of the family. Thomas Fullwood was a screw maker employing six people and his ability and desire to purchase a vault is some indication perhaps of his wealth and standing in the community. John Carter and his wife Mary were associated with the brewing industry and owned several properties in the town, clear indications of the wealth that enabled them to buy a vault (see Chapter 6). The Carter and Fullwood grave memorials each list three members of the family, mother, father and son, and it is possible that other members of the family could be interred in the same vault. However, the fact that the vaults were in the burial ground and not in the churchyard is perhaps an indication that, although wealthy enough to buy a vault, they did not have the social standing to own one in the churchyard. Conversely, it could just be because the churchyard was full.

At St Martin's, the vaults were built not only for the wealthy ironmaster and brass founder, but also for a chemist and a saddler, demonstrating that the acquisition of a vault was not just reserved for the very rich (Brickley *et al* 2006) but for those who, perhaps like the Carter and Fullwood families, had become successful entrepreneurs. Unfortunately, the excavations could not confirm that other burials in the vault were related to the relevant families, so these vaults may have been more of a public facility for people to buy spaces in.

The five-year period (1850–1855) detailed above, when the churchwarden provided details of those who were buried in the burial ground, enables us look more closely at a few of the interments. Of the 27 names listed as buried in a vault within the burial ground during that time, all except two were local and the majority were found to have lived in the streets close to the centre of the town, suggesting that they were mainly drawn from the working classes. However, the fact that they had a vault burial could suggest that they had sufficient means to afford it, an indication perhaps of some degree of success in their working lives.

Eight of the vault burials were of children under two years old, with four of those under six months, an indication of the high infant mortality rate at the time. It is perhaps interesting that the families of these children could afford a vault burial. Families at that time might experience the loss of several young children which would, for some, constitute considerable expense, so this might show something of the esteem that they felt for their children, however young.

The parish burial register itself provided some useful information about local people: notably Thomas Stoner Simkiss of Waterloo Road, who died aged 77 in February 1868, and Mary Stoner Simkiss, who was 81 when she died in December 1871, both of whom were described as 'Roman Catholics', and it was noted that they did not have a service. This could be considered somewhat unusual for a Roman Catholic burial in an Anglican burial ground, but can be explained by examining the older records where, in the 1780s, other members of the Stoner Simkiss family were listed, indicating the presence of a family vault or tomb. In addition, up to the 1740s several burials were annotated with 'Papist', including one George Brown, a Papist Priest who was buried in

January 1713. At that time St Peter's was the only burial ground available in Wolverhampton so this would account for their presence, and demonstrate some degree of religious tolerance at the time in relation to burials.

From the 1500s until 2002, St Peter's Collegiate Church provided the town with a place to bury their dead. From the 1850s, when government legislation restricted burial in churchyards, numbers fell dramatically to only 120 between 1862 and 1899, and to 19 between 1900 and 1937. It is likely that many of those since 1900, together with the few others that took place in the ensuing years and that are recorded at the church, were caskets of ashes placed in existing vaults.

This excavation of a small part of the overflow burial ground of St Peter's Church, Wolverhampton, has provided an in-depth study of people who lived and worked in the town during the 19th century. The results have enabled comparisons to be made with similar excavations in the Midlands, thus contributing to the increasing pool of knowledge about the lives of the people, together with the ritual associated with their demise. The most detailed information has been recovered from the sketetal remains themselves, which belie the occupation and lifestyle of those buried at the church. Osteoarchaeological analysis has highlighted the physical effects of living and working in an industrial city – and the stark differences in health and occupation, between rural and urban dwellers.

Abbreviations

BUFAU   Birmingham University Field Archaeology Unit
OED   Oxford English Dictionary
Staffordshire RO Staffordshire Record Office

Bibliography

Adams, J, and Cherrington, R, 2002 *Excavations at St Martin's Churchyard 2001. Post-excavation assessment and updated project design*. BUFAU Report No. 798

Allbutt 1898 cited in the Oxford English Dictionary

Arabaolaza, I, Ponce, P, and Boyston, A, 2005 *St Peter's Collegiate Church, Wolverhampton: report on the human skeletal remains*. Biological Anthropology Research Centre Report 6. University of Bradford

Aufderheide, A C, and Rodríguez-Martín, C, 1998 *The Cambridge Encyclopedia of Human Paleopathology*. Cambridge: Cambridge University Press

Barnsby, G J, 1980 *Social Conditions in the Black Country 1800–1900*. Wolverhampton: Integrated Publishing Services

Barnsby, G J, 1987 *A History of Housing in Wolverhampton 1750–1975*. Wolverhampton: Integrated Publishing Services (reprint of pre-1975 edition)

Bartley, P, 1996 *The Changing Role of Women 1815–1914*. London: Hodder & Stoughton

Bass, W M, 1987 *Human Osteology: a laboratory and field manual*. Missouri: Missouri Archaeological Society (3rd edition)

Behrensmayer, A K, 1978 Taphonomic and ecologic information from bone weathering, *Paleobiology*, 4, 150–62

Berry, A C, and Berry, R J, 1967 Epigenetic variation in the human cranium, *Journal of Anatomy*, 101, 361–79

Blair, J, and Pyrah, C (eds), 1996 *Church Archaeology: research directions for the future*, CBA Research Report 104. York: Council for British Archaeology

Boocock, P, Roberts, C, and Manchester, K, 1995 Maxillary sinusitis in medieval Chichester, England, *American Journal of Physical Anthropology*, 98, 483–95

Boore E, 1998 Burial vaults and coffin furniture in the West Country, in M Cox (ed) 1998, 67–84

Bowman, J E, MacLaughlin, S M, and Scheue, J L, 1993 A study of documentary and skeletal evidence relating to 18th and 19th century crypt burials in the City of London: The St. Bride's Project, *American Journal of Physical Anthropology*, Suppl 16, 60

Boyle, A, 2004 What price compromise? Archaeological investigations at St Bartholomew's Church, Penn, Wolverhampton, *Church Archaeology*, 5 and 6, 69–79

Boylston, A, and Roberts, C, 2004 The Roman inhumations, in M Dawson (ed) 2004, 322–70

Brickley, M, Buteux, S, with Adams, J, and Cherrington, R, 2006 *St Martin's Uncovered: investigations in the churchyard of St. Martin's-in-the-Bull-Ring, Birmingham 2001*. Oxford: Oxbow

Brickley, M, and Miles, A, with Stainer, H, 1999 *The Cross Bones Burial Ground, Redcross Way Southwark, London: archaeological excavations (1991–1998) for the London Underground Limited Jubilee Line Extension Project*. MoLAS Monograph 3. London: Museum of London Archaeology Service

Brickley, M, and McKinley, J (eds) 2004 *Guidelines to the Standards for Recording Human Remains*. IFA Technical paper no 7. BABAO, Southampton University

Brickley, M, and Smith, M, 2006 Culturally determined patterns of violence: biological anthropological investigations at a historic urban cemetery, *American Anthropologist*, 108, No. 1, 173

Brooks, S T, and Suchey, J M, 1990 Skeletal age determination based on the os pubis: a comparison of the Acsádi-Nemeskéri and Suchey-Brooks Methods, *Human Evolution*, 5, 227–38

Brothwell, D R, 1981 *Digging up Bones*. London: British Museum (Natural History) (3rd edition)

Buikstra, J E, and Ubelaker, D H (eds), 1994 *Standards for Data Collection from Human Skeletal Remains. Proceedings of a seminar at the Field Museum of Natural History*. Indianapolis: Arkansas Archaeological Survey Research Seminar Series No. 44

Bush, H, and Zvelebil, M (eds), 1991 *Health in Past Societies: biocultural interpretations of human skeletal remains in archaeological contexts.* Oxford: BAR Publishing

Cassell's Domestic Dictionary: an enclopaedia for the household 1884. London: Cassell, Petter, Galpin and Co

Chadwick, O, 1966 *The Victorian Church.* London: Adams and Charles

Children's Employment Commission. British Parliamentary Papers, Vol XV

Cook, G H, 1959 *English Collegiate Churches of the Middle Ages.* London: Phoenix House

Coates, G, and Litherland, S, 1996 *An Archaeological Salvage Recording and Watching Brief at the University of Wolverhampton, Wolverhampton, West Midlands.* BUFAU Report 417

Coates, G, and Neilson, C, 2002 *Excavations in Advance of the Extension to the Harrison Learning Centre, University of Wolverhampton, West Midlands. Post-excavation Assessment and Updated Project Design.* BUFAU Report 846

Cockin, T, 2000 *The Staffordshire Encyclopaedia.* Stoke on Trent: Malthouse Press

Cox, M (ed), 1998 *Grave Concerns: death and burial in England 1700–1850*, CBA Research Report 113. York: Council for British Archaeology

Curl, J S, 1972 *Victorian Celebration of Death.* Newton Abott: David and Charles

Curl, J S, 2000 *The Victorian Celebration of Death.* Stroud: Sutton Publishing

Darlington, J, forthcoming *Excavations at Stafford Castle* Vol. 2

Davidoff, L, and Hall, C, 1987 *Family Fortunes: men and women of the English middle class.* London: Hutchinson (repr. Routledge 1992)

Dawson, M (ed), 2004 *Archaeology in the Bedford region,* British Archaeological Reports, Brit Ser 373. Oxford: BAR Publishing

Dias, G, and Tayles, N, 1997 'Abscess cavity' – a misnomer, *International Journal of Osteoarchaeology,* 7, 548–54

Dickens, C, (1868) 1933 *The Uncommercial Traveller,* in *Barnaby Rudge.* London: Hazell, Watson and Viney

Duckworth, T, 1980 *Lecture Notes on Orthopaedics and Fractures.* Oxford: Blackwell scientific publications

Edlin, H L, 1949 *Woodland Crafts in Britain.* London: Batsford

Finnegan, M, 1978 Non-metric variation of the infracranial skeleton, *Journal of Anatomy,* 125, 23–37

Flanders, J, 2003 *The Victorian House. Domestic life fron childbirth to deathbed.* London: Harper Collins

Fox, L, 1947 Coventry's heritage, *The Coventry Evening Telegraph.* Coventry

Gale, R, and Cutler, D, 2000 *Plants in Archaeology: identification manual of vegetative plant materials used in Europe and the southern Mediterranean to c. 1500.* Otley: Westbury and Royal Botanic Gardens, Kew

Goose, D H, 1981 Changes in human face breadth since the mediaeval period in Britain, *Archives of Oral Biology,* 26, 757–8

Hall-Matthews, J C B 1993 *The Collegiate Church of St Peter, Wolverhampton.* Much Wenlock: RJL Smith

Harding, V, 1998 Burial on the margin: distance and discrimination in early modern London, in M Cox (ed) 1998

Hillson, S, 1996 *Dental Anthropology.* Cambridge: Cambridge University Press

Hillson, S W, Waldron, H A, Martin, L A, and Owen-Smith, B, 1999 The bones from Benjamin Franklin's house at Craven Street, London, *American Journal of Physical Anthropology* Annual Meeting Issue

Hooke, D, 1986 Wolverhampton: the town and its monastery, in D Hooke and T R Slater 1986

Hooke, D, and Slater, T R, 1986 *Anglo Saxon Wolverhampton. The town and its monastery.* Wolverhampton: Libraries and Community Services Division. Wolverhampton Borough Council

Hopkins, E, 1979 *A Social History of the English Working Classes 1815–1945.* London: Hodder & Stoughton

Horne, R H, 1843 The Iron Trade and other Manufacturers. *Children's Employment Commission,* 561–97

Isçan, M Y (ed), 1989 *Age Markers in the Human Skeleton.* Springfield (IL): Charles C Thomas

Isçan, M Y, Loth, S R, and Wright, R K, 1984 Age estimation from the rib by phase analysis: white males, *Journal of Forensic Sciences*, 29, 1094–104

Isçan, M Y, Loth, S R, and Wright, R K, 1985 Age estimation from the rib by phase analysis: white females, *Journal of Forensic Sciences*, 30, 853–63

Jalland, P, 1996 *Death in a Victorian Family*. Oxford: Oxford University Press

Jurmain, R, 1999 *Stories from the Skeleton: behavioural reconstruction in human osteology*. Amsterdam: Gordon and Breach.

Kiple, K F (ed), 1993 *The Cambridge World History of Human Disease*. Cambridge: Cambridge University Press

Krakowicz, R, and Rudge, A, 2002 *Masshouse Circus, Birmingham City Centre*. Birmingham Archaeology Report No. 923

Krapp, K, and Longe, J L, *c* 2001 *The Gale Encyclopaedia of Alternative Medicine*. Detroit; London: Gale Group

Krogman, W M, and Isçan, M Y, 1986 *The Human Skeleton in Forensic Medicine*. Springfield, Illinois: Charles C Thomas (2nd edition)

Lewis, M, Roberts, C, and Manchester, K, 1995 Comparative study of the prevalence of maxillary sinusitis in later medieval urban and rural populations in northern England, *American Journal of Physical Anthropology*, 98, 497–506

Lewis, M, 1999 *The Impact of Urbanisation and Industrialisation in Medieval and Post-Medieval Britain. An assessment of the morbidity and mortality of non-adult skeletons from cemeteries of two urban and two rural sites in England (AD 850–1859)*. Unpublished PhD thesis, University of Bradford

Lewis, M, 2002 *Urbanisation and Child Health in Medieval and Post-Medieval England: an assessment of the morbidity and mortality of non-adult skeletons from the cemeteries of two urban and two rural sites in England (AD 850–1859)*, British Archaeological Reports, Brit Ser 339. Oxford: BAR Publishing

Lincoln, W A, 1986 *World Woods in Colour*. London: Stobart and Sons

Litten, J, 1991 *The English Way of Death: the common funeral since 1450*. London: Robert Hale

Lovejoy, C O, Meindl, R S, Pryzbeck, T R, and Mensfort, R P, 1985 Chronological metamorphosis of the auricular surface of the ilium: a new method for the determination of age at death, *American Journal of Physical Anthropology*, 68, 15–28

Luther, F, 1993 A cephalometric comparison of medieval skulls with a modern population, *European Journal of Orthodontics*, 15, 315–25

McKenna, J, 1992 *In the Midst of Life*. Birmingham: Birmingham Library Service

Mander, G P, and Tildesley, N W, 1960 *A History of Wolverhampton to the Early Nineteenth Century*. Wolverhampton: Wolverhampton Corporation

Mays, S, 1998 *The Archaeology of Human Bones*. Routledge: London

Meindl, R S, and Lovejoy, C O, 1985 Ectocranial suture closure: a revised method for the determination of skeletal age at death based on the lateral-anterior sutures, *American Journal of Physical Anthropology*, 68, 57–66

Meindl, R S, and Lovejoy, C O, 1989 Age changes in the pelvis: implications for paleodemography, in M Y Isçan (ed) 1989, 137–68

Mitchell, A, 1974 *A Field Guide to the Trees of Britain and Northern Europe*. London: Collins

Mitchell, J, 1842 *Children's Employment Commission* 1st Report Mines

Molleson, T, and Cox, M, with Waldron, A H, and Whittaker, D K, 1993 *The Spitalfields Project: Vol. 2 The Anthropology: the middling sort*, CBA Research Report 86. York: Council for British Archaeology

Moorrees, C F A, Fanning, E A, and Hunt, E E, 1963a Formation and resorption of three deciduous teeth in children, *American Journal of Physical Anthropology*, 21, 205–13

Moorrees, C F A, Fanning, E A, and Hunt, E E, 1963b Age variation of formation stages for ten permanent teeth, *Journal of Dental Research*, 42, 1490–502

Morley, J, 1971 *Death, Heaven and the Victorians*. London: Studio Vista

Neilson, C, and Coates, G, 2002 *Excavations in Advance of the Extension to the Harrison Learning Centre, University of Wolverhampton, West Midlands 2001. Post-excavation assessment*. BUFAU Project No. 846

O'Brien, E, and Roberts, C, 1996 Archaeological study of church cemeteries: past, present and future, in J Blair and C Pyrah (eds) 1996

Ogden, A R, Boylston A, Vaughan, T, 2005 Tallow Hill Cemetery, Worcester: the importance of detailed study of post-medieval graveyards, in S Zakrzewski and M Clegg (eds) 2005, 51–8

Ortner, D J, 2003 *Identification of Pathological Conditions in Human Skeletal Remains*. London: Academic Press (2nd edition)

Orton, I, 1976 *Maps of Wolverhampton*. Wolverhampton: Wolverhampton Public Libraries

Owen, I, 1889 Reports of the Collective Investigation Committee of the British Medical Association. Geographical distribution of rickets, acute and subacute rheumatism, chorea, cancer, and unrinary calculus in the British Islands, *British Medical Journal*, 1, 113–16

Patrick, C, 2001 *The Churchyard of St Philips Cathedral, Birmingham*. BUFAU Report No. 701

Price, J, 1832 *A Brief Narrative of the Events Relative to the Cholera at Bilston, in the Year 1832*. Bilston: George Price

Quetel, C, 1986 *La Mal de Naples: histoire de la syphilis*. Paris: Seghers. Translated Braddock, J, and Pike, B, 1990 *History of Syphilis*. London: Polity Press with Basil Blackwell

Rackham, O, 1986 *The History of the Countryside*. London: Dent

Rátkai, S, in preparation The pottery, in J Darlington forthcoming

Rawlinson, R, 1849 *Report to the General Board of Health on a preliminary inquiry into the sewerage, drainage, and supply of water, and the sanitary condition of the inhabitants of the borough of Wolverhampton, and the townships of Bilston, Willenhall, and Wednesfield*. Public Health Act. London: W Clowes and Sons for HMSO

Resnick, D, Shapiro, R, Wiesner, K, Niwayama, G, Utsinger, P and Shaul, S, 1978 Diffuse idiopathic skeletal hyperostosis (DISH) [Ankylosing hyperostosis of Rotes-Querol], *Seminars in Arthritis and Rheumatism*, 7, 153–87

Resnick, D, and Niwayama, G, 1995 *Diagnosis of Bone and Joint Disorders*. London: W B Saunders (3rd edition)

Richardson, R, 1987 *Death, Dissection and the Destitute*. London: Routledge and Kegan Paul

Riley, N, 1991 *Gifts for Good Children, Part 1: The History of Children's China 1790–1890*. Ilminster: Richard Dennis

Roberts, C, Boylston, A, Buckley, L, Chamberlain, A, and Murphy, E, 1998 Rib lesions and tuberculosis: the palaeopathological evidence, *Tubercle and Lung Disease*, 79 (1), 55–60

Roberts, C, and Cox, M, 2003 *Health & Disease in Britain: from prehistory to the present day*. Stroud: Sutton Publishing

Roberts, C, and Manchester, K, 1995 *The Archaeology of Disease*. Stroud: Alan Sutton (2nd edition)

Robson, G, 2002 *Dark Satanic Mills? Religion and irreligion in Birmingham and the Black Country*. Carlisle: Paternoster Press

Rogers, J, and Waldron, T, 1995 *A Field Guide to Joint Disease in Archaeology*. West Sussex: John Wiley & Sons

Roper, J, 1969 *Trades and Professions in Wolverhampton, 1802: a directory compiled from the 1802 rate book*. Wolverhampton Local History Pamphlet – No. 3. Wolverhampton

Rothschild, B, and Woods, R, 1991 Spondyloarthropathy: erosive arthritis in representative defleshed bones, *American Journal of Physical Anthropology*, 85, 125–34

Shaw, M, 2001 *University of Wolverhampton, Extension to Harrison Learning Centre. Brief for Archaeological Work*. Wolverhampton City Council

Scheuer, L, and Black, S, 2000 *Developmental Juvenile Osteology*. London: Academic Press

Scheuer, L, and Black, S, 2004 *The Juvenile Skeleton*. Oxford: Elsevier Academic Press

Showell, W, 1885 *Dictionary of Birmingham*. Birmingham: Cornish

Slater, T R, 1986 Wolverhampton: central place to medieval borough, in D Hooke and T R Slater 1986

Stallard, R, n.d. *Wolverhampton Hospitals Heritage*. Wombourne: Wombourne Printers

Stewart, T D (ed), 1970 *Personal Identification in Mass Disasters*. Washington (DC): National Museum of Natural History, Smithsonian Institute

Stewart, T D, 1979 *Essentials of Forensic Anthropology: especially as developed in the United States*. Springfield (IL): Charles C Thomas

Stuart-Macadam, P, 1987 Porotic hyperostosis: new evidence to support the anaemia theory, *American Journal of Physical Anthropology*, 74, 521–6

Stuart-Macadam, P, 1991 Anaemia in Roman Britain: Poundbury Camp, in H Bush and M Zvelebil (eds) 1991, 101–13

Stuart-Macadam, P, 1992 Porotic hyperostosis: a new perspective, *American Journal of Physical Anthropology*, 87, 39–47

Sundick, R I, 1978 Human skeletal growth and age determination, *Homo*, 29, 228–49

Tancred, T, 1843 *Midland Mining Company 1st Report, South Staffs*

Todd, T W, 1921a Age changes in the pubic bone. I: the male white pubis, *American Journal of Physical Anthropology*, 3, 285–334

Todd, T W, 1921b Age changes in the pubic bone. III: the pubis of the white female. IV: the pubis of the female white-negro hybrid, *American Journal of Physical Anthropology*, 4, 1–70

Tomes, J, 1851 *Instructions on the Use and Management of Artificial Teeth*. London

Trotter, M, 1970 Estimation of stature form intact long limb bones, in T D Stewart (ed) 1970, 71–4

Ubelaker, D H, 1989 *Human Skeletal Remains*. Washington (DC): Taraxacum Press (2nd edition)

Upton, C, 1998 *A History of Wolverhampton*. Chichester: Phillimore

VCH 1970 *The Victoria History of the Counties of England. A History of the County of Stafford, Vol III*, ed M W Greenslade. London: Oxford University Press for the University of London, Institute of Historical Research

Waldron, T, 1985 DISH at Merton Priory: evidence for a 'new' occupational disease? *British Medical Journal*, 291, 1762–3

Waldron, T, 1994 *Counting the Dead: the epidemiology of skeletal populations*. Chichester: John Wiley and Sons

Watt, S, 2001 *Extension to the Harrison Learning Centre, University of Wolverhampton: an archaeological desk-based assessment*. BUFAU Report 828

Witkin, A, 1997 *The cutting edge: aspects of amputations in the late 18th and early 19th century*. Unpublished University of Sheffield and University of Bradford M.Sc. thesis

Wohl, A S, 1983 *Endangered Lives: Public Health in Victorian Britain*. Dent: London

Wolverhampton Borough Council Library 1993 *Mapping the Past – Wolverhampton 1577–1986*. Metropolitan Borough of Wolverhampton and Information Services Division

Wood, R, and Woodward, J (eds), 1984 *Urban Disease and Mortality in Nineteenth-Century England*. London: Batsford Academic and Educational

Woodforde, J, 1995 *A History of Vanity*. Stroud: Sutton Publishing

Zakrzewski , S, and Clegg, M (eds), 2005 *Proceedings of the Fifth Annual Conference of the British Association for Biological Anthropology and Osteoarchaeology*. British Archaeological Reports, Int Ser 133. Oxford: BAR Publishing

Trade Directories

The Birmingham Directory 1787
Wolverhampton Directory 1805–7, 1858 and 1869
Commercial Directory for 1818–20
Staffordshire Directory 1818
Smart's Trade Directory 1827
White's Staffordshire Directory 1834
Bridgens Directory of the Borough of Wolverhampton 1838
Robson's Birmingham and Sheffield Directory of Birmingham, Coventry, Dudley and Wolverhampton 1839
Post Office Directory of London Birmingham with Warwickshire & part of South Staffordshire 1845
Kelly's Directory of Birmingham, Staffordshire and Worcestershire 1850
Slater's Directory of Birmingham and District 1851
Melville & Co's Directory & Gazatteer for Wolverhampton & Neighbourhood 1851
Post Office Directory of Birmingham, Staffordshire, Warwickshire and Worcestershire 1860

Primary Sources

Census Returns for 1841, 1851, 1861, and 1871
Rates for 1792
Probate will of John Carter of Wolverhampton, beer retailer 9/9/1863 (Wolverhampton Archives ref.: DX195/8)
Requisitions on title: trustees under the will of Mary Carter, deceased....1877 (Wolverhampton Archives ref.: CMB/WOL/D/J40/6,7)
Abstract of title: of trustees of late Mrs. Mary Carter and Mr. William Potts to the dwelling houses and premises in Canal Street, 1877 (Wolverhampton Archives ref.: CMB/WOL/D/J40/6,7)
Mortgage: Mary Carter of Wolverhampton, victualler, 6/1/1868 (Wolverhampton Archives ref.: DX195/16)
Conveyance: Mary Carter of Wolverhampton, widow (Wolverhampton Archives ref.: DX195/17)

Borough of Wolverhampton – Report of the General Purposes Committee to the Council, 20/12/1899

St Peter's Burial Records 1818–1865

Death certificates for John Carter, Thomas Watwood Carter and Thomas Fullwood

Wolverhampton Photographic Society photographs of Charles Street

Cholera – Staffordshire Study Book II, Wolverhampton Public Libraries

The Collegiate Church of St Peter Wolverhampton – Guide Book

Staffordshire Adveriser 1832

Wolverhampton Chronicle 9th December 1812, 9th February 1843, 26th July 1843, 23rd August 1843, 26th January 1848, 9 February 1848, 1st March 1848

Maps

1750   Isaac Taylor map of Wolverhampton
1788   Godson's map of Wolverhampton
1827   Map of the town of Wolverhampton
1842   Tithe map
1852   Health of the Towns map
1871   Plan of Wolverhampton
1889   First Edition Ordnance Survey map
1901   Stephens and Mackintosh Business map
1902   Second Edition Ordnance Survey map
1919   Third Edition Ordnance Survey map
1938   Ordnance Survey map

Internet References

www.findarticles.com – Gale Encyclopaedia of Alternative Medicines

http://home.clara.net/rod.beavon/tipton.htm

www.localhistory.scit.wlv.ac.uk

www.localhistory.scit.wlv.ac.uk/articles/RoyalHospital

www.localhistory.scit.wlv.ac.uk/articles/Jennings/jennings.htm

www.oed.com – Oxford English Dictionary

http://pers-www.wlv.ac.uk/~in2021/oldwlv.htm

www.scit.wlv.ac.uk/local/victorian

www.swan.ac.uk/teaching

http://www.tiscali.co.uk/reference/encyclopaedia/hutchinson/m0021631.html

www.tiscali/myweb.co.uk/poetrypages/photo

Glossary of Palaeopathological Terminology

(definitions are adapted from the 27th edition of Dorland's Illustrated Medical Dictionary published in 1988 by W B Saunders Co)

Abrasion	The wearing away of a structure such as a tooth
Abscess	A localised collection of pus in a confined space
Acromioclavicular	The joint between the collar bone and the shoulder blade
Aetiology	The factors that cause a disease
Agenesis	Absence of an organ, eg as a result of embryonic development
Alveolar bone	The bone surrounding the teeth
Ankylose(is)	Fusion of a joint
Ante mortem	An event which took place before death occurred
Anterior	Situated in the front of the body
Antrum(al)	The sinus chamber (eg in the maxilla surrounding the nasal region)
Apical	Located at the apex, eg the end of the tooth root
Apophyseal	The joints that link the vertebrae of the spine
Appendicular	The appendages of the skeleton, namely the upper and lower limbs
Attrition	Wear on the teeth in the course of normal use
Auricular	The articular surface on the ilium (for the sacro-iliac joint) which is shaped like an ear
Avulsion	The ripping or tearing away of a part
Axial	The axial skeleton consists of the cranium and torso
Bevelling	A slanting edge
Bicondylar	The distance between the mandibular condyles
Buccal	Surface of the tooth nearest the cheek
Calcaneus	Heel bone
Calculus	Tartar
Caries	Cavities in the teeth
Cariogenic	Conducive to the production of caries
Cloaca	A hole in the bone allowing pus to escape
Compensatory eruption	The tendency of a tooth to continue to erupt in adulthood so that the surfaces remain in occlusion despite the tooth wear
Congenital	Conditions which are present at birth, regardless of their causation.
Cortical defect	A depression in the surface of the bone due to muscle pull
Costochondral	The junction between the bone of a rib and its cartilage
Costovertebral	The joints between the ribs and the vertebrae of the spine
Deciduous	Teeth from the first dentition which are shed during childhood
Diaphysis	Shaft of a long bone before the ends have fused
Disarticulated	Bone which is separated from the rest of the skeleton usually as a result of post-mortem processes
Distal	Position on the dental arch further from median line of jaw
Eburnated	Polished or burnished
Endocranium	The inner table of the skull
Enthesophyte	A bony outgrowth at the insertion of a tendon or ligament on bone
Epiphysis (eal)	The expanded end of a long bone which is separated from the shaft by cartilage during growth
Erosion	Progressive loss of the hard substance of a tooth by chemical processes
External auditory meatus	The bony structure surrounding the ear
External occipital protuberance	The bony structure which protrudes on the posterior cranium
Flexor	Any muscle which flexes a joint
Foramen	A natural opening or passage through the bone
Gonial	Pertaining to the lower jaw

Granuloma	A collection of inflammatory cells representing a chronic inflammatory process
Haematoma	A localised collection of blood in an organ or tissue
Herniation	The abnormal protrusion of a body structure through a defect in muscle or bone
Hypertrophic	Increased amount of bone
Hypoplasia	Incomplete or underdevelopment of an organ or tissue
Interproximal	Between adjacent surface, eg of the teeth
Lambdoid	The junction between the parietal and occipital bones
Lingual	Surface of tooth nearest to the tongue
Lytic	A destructive process in bone
Macroscopic	Examined with the naked eye
Mandible(ular)	Lower jaw
Masticatory	Concerned with the process of chewing food
Maxilla(ry)	Upper jaw
Mesial	Surface of tooth nearest to the median plane of dental arch
Metastatic	The transfer of disease from one organ to another
Metopic	The suture in the middle of the frontal bone which normally closes in early childhood
Microstructure	The microscopic appearance of the tissues
Morphological	Concerned with shape
Mucosa	The lining of an orifice such as the mouth or nose
Neoplasia	Any new and abnormal growth
Oro-antral fistula	A pathological opening between the mouth and the sinus chamber
Orthognathic	Characterised by minimal protrusion of the mandible, the opposite of prognathism
Os acromiale	Failure of the top of the acromial process of the scapula to fuse with the acromion at the normal time in adolescence
Ossicle	A small bone
Ossification	The conversion of fibrous tissue into a bony structure
Osteitis	Inflammation of a bone
Osteology	The scientific study of the bones
Osteophyte	A bony excrescence
Overjet	Horizontal overlap (eg of the upper jaw)
Peri mortem	An event occurring around the time of death
Periodontal	Pertaining to the tissues which support the teeth
Periodontitis	Inflammation of the tissues surrounding the teeth
Periosteum	A specialised connective tissue covering all the bones of the body
Periostitis	Inflammation of the periosteum
Plaque	A soft, thin film of mucin, food debris and epithelial cells deposited on the teeth
Platycnemia	Medio-lateral flattening of the shaft of the tibia
Platymeria	Antero-posterior flattening of the shaft of the femur
Postcranial	The part of the skeleton below the cranium or skull
Preauricular	Situated in front of the auricular surface of the ilium
Proximal	Part of the body closer to any point of reference
Pubic symphysis	The joint between the two pelvic bones at the front in the midline
Sacralisation	Fusion of the fifth lumbar vertebra to the first sacral vertebra
Sacroiliac	The joint between the sacrum and the *os coxa* or pelvic bone
Sagittal	In the mid-line of the cranium or postcranial skeleton
Sclerosing	A thickening of the bone which is most clearly seen on X-ray
Sesamoid bone	A small nodular bone embedded in a tendon or joint capsule
Shear	A force caused by an opposite but parallel sliding moion of the planes of an object
Spina bifida occulta	A defect of the bony spinal canal (usually seen in the sacrum) without protrusion of the spinal cord
Spondylolysis	Separation of the body and neural arch of the vertebra
Sternoclavicular	The joint between the breast bone and the collar bone
Subchondral	The bone lying beneath the cartilage of an articular surface
Subluxation	Partial dislocation

Subpubic	The angle formed by the joint between the two pubic bones in the midline of the body anteriorly
Supernumerary	In addition to the normal number
Suppurative	Producing pus
Suture	Type of fibrous joint where opposing surfaces are closely united
Symphysis	A fibro-cartilaginous joint in the midline of the body
Synovial	A very mobile joint such as the hip, knee, elbow, etc. Also the smaller joints in the body, eg in fingers and toes
Torsion	The process of twisting or rotating around an axis
Treponemal	caused by a bacterium of the Spirochete family. Diseases caused by treponemes include syphilis, yaws and pinta
Visceral	The internal surface of the ribs
Wormian	Small additional bones within the sutures of the cranium

APPENDIX 1

Identifying and Scoring Periodontal Disease in Skeletal Material

A R Ogden

Biological Anthropology Research Centre, Department of Archaeological Sciences,
University of Bradford, BD7 1DP, UK

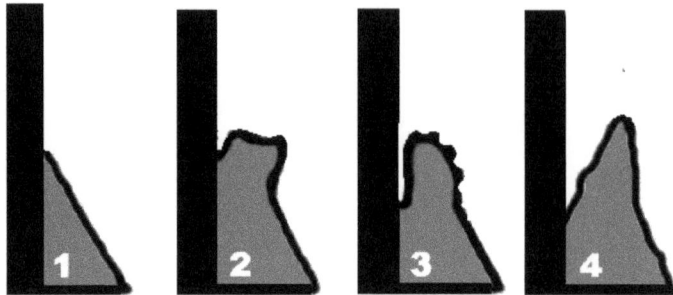

1 Alveolar margin meets tooth at a knife-edged acute angle (No disease).
2 Alveolar margin is blunted and flat-topped (Mild periodontitis).
3 Alveolar margin is rounded, with a trough 2–4mm depth between tooth and alveolus (Moderate periodontitis).
4 Alveolar margin is ragged, with an irregular trough >5mm depth between tooth and alveolus (Severe periodontitis).

NB The length of root exposed is irrelevant, as this may be simply a function of compensatory eruption.

www.ingramcontent.com/pod-product-compliance
Lightning Source LLC
Chambersburg PA
CBHW061008030426
42334CB00033B/3402